HOLISTIC HEALTH
for **ADOLESCENTS**

HOLISTIC HEALTH
for ADOLESCENTS

How yoga, aromatherapy,
teas, and more
can help you get
and stay well

Nada Milosavljevic, MD, JD

W. W. Norton & Company

Independent Publishers Since 1923

New York • London

Important Note: *Holistic Health for Adolescents* is intended to provide general information on the subject of health and well-being; it is not a substitute for medical or psychological treatment and may not be relied upon for purposes of diagnosing or treating any illness. Please seek out the care of a professional healthcare provider if you are pregnant, nursing, or experiencing symptoms of any potentially serious condition.

For information about permission to reproduce selections from this book, write to Permissions, W. W. Norton & Company, Inc., 500 Fifth Avenue, New York, NY 10110.

For information about special discounts for bulk purchases, please contact W. W. Norton Special Sales at specialsales@wwnorton.com or 800-233-4830

Manufacturing by Edwards Brothers Molloy
Production manager: Christine Critelli

Library of Congress Cataloging-in-Publication Data

Milosavljevic, Nada, Medical doctor.
Holistic health for adolescents/ Nada Milosavljevic.
First edition.
p. cm.
   Includes bibliographical references and index.
         ISBN: 978-0-393-71114-1 (pbk.)
1. Adolescent psychopathology.
   2. Teenagers—Diseases—Alternative treatment. 3. Holistic medicine.
RJ503 .M554 2016
616.8900835—dc23

                                                              2016002830

W. W. Norton & Company, Inc., 500 Fifth Avenue, New York, N.Y. 10110
www.wwnorton.com

W. W. Norton & Company Ltd., Castle House, 75/76 Wells Street, London W1T 3QT

1 2 3 4 5 6 7 8 9 0

TO THE HIGH SCHOOL STUDENTS WHO PARTICIPATED
IN THE INTEGRATIVE HEALTH PROGRAM:

You taught me so much more than I could ever have shared with you. With gratitude and heartfelt thanks for inspiring me with your resilience and spirit. And for teaching me the school bell was not the fire alarm.

—"Dr. M"

Contents

////////////////////

PREFACE

//////////////////////////

In December 2010, I became director of the Integrative Health Program at Massachusetts General Hospital. Since that time, I've been promoting novel and effective approaches for improving mental health among teens. Teaching adolescents how to understand, manage, and, in some cases, overcome their mental health problems has given me great joy and deep satisfaction. There's nothing more rewarding than seeing kids improve their lives dramatically with holistic therapies, like those included in this book. With these tools, adolescents feel empowered and better equipped for many challenges they may face. In the following pages, I discuss many of the therapies I've shared with students at several high school clinics in the Boston area.

There's quite a lot of work and preparation involved in assessing kids who are facing challenging emotional circumstances in their lives. So, even though I feel very lucky to be doing what I'm doing, I can sometimes get caught up in details and forget to be grateful for all that I've learned and how it can be helpful to others. Luckily, once in a while, something wonderful happens that serves as a powerful reminder.

In 2014, on an early spring morning, I was walking to a meeting about a mile from where I work at Massachusetts General Hospital. On my way, I went to get something hot to drink at a little café in the neighborhood. Standing in line surrounded by shiny display counters and the hum of happy customers, I was startled to hear somebody addressing me directly. "Dr. Nada. Dr. Nada!" I heard over my shoulder. The person calling me was Laura, a high school patient of mine from 2011. "Hey guys," she said, including her coworkers in this conversation. "This is Dr. Nada. She's the doctor who helped me when I was stressing out in high school. I told you I used acupuncture when I was stressed out about job interviews. Remember?" Three or four of her friends gathered next to me and took an impromptu break to hear Laura's stories, and I stood quietly as she described her experience and positive benefits from integrative treatments. I had always told my patients that doctor-patient confidentiality was very important, but Laura wasn't too worried about keeping her therapy sessions under wraps at this point.

I was surprised and heartened by Laura's lack of reserve concerning her experience in my clinic. One of the largest and most enduring obstacles to kids seeking and receiving treatment for mental health issues (and adults too, for that matter) is the stigma that's often associated with it. Yet here Laura was, actively inviting people to listen to her experiences, and then encouraging them to seek the same kind of help if they needed it. Laura had certainly come a long way from the girl who could barely take tests and felt challenged in social situations because she was so nervous. Her nervousness had stemmed from a lot of different sources, including being part of a family with significant financial problems and parental discord. When she came to my clinic, her own skepticism about integrative treatments was overcome by her need for some solution. I was glad she trusted me, gave acupuncture and acupressure a try, and then later found the confidence to apply these methods on her own when she needed them.

Looking back at myself in my early 20s, I would never have been as enthusiastic as Laura about any type of holistic medicine. Although I didn't know it back then, I was naturally inclined to be an adherent of evidence-based medicine. Treatments like acupuncture, yoga, and music therapy seemed like anecdotal folkore. But, after many different experiences and surprises in my career and education, I came to see that these kinds of therapies could be very effective—in terms of both costs and outcomes. And the evidence is accumulating year after year that we can—and should—use these therapies when appropriate. But it took many years for me to understand this.

/////

MY FIRST CAREER was in law. And at the age of 24, my first big job was as an associate attorney at a law firm that specialized in intellectual property protection for pharmaceutical firms and research institutes. How I became a lawyer stretches back to my childhood. Although I grew up in the United States, almost all of my family was from Serbia or Croatia, which were both part of the former Yugoslavia. I had wonderful experiences visiting my family in eastern Europe, but while there, I noticed a sort of sadness in the country, due, from what I understood at the time, to a lack of hope. Any visitor, even a young one, could see that the economy was stifled. On one hand, the burden of communism constricted people's lives and limited their freedom. If you did have freedom to create, your creations (be they technical, artistic, or financial) were not well protected. Thus, creativity and entrepreneurship were stifled and the progress that depends on that creativity could not take place. People's lives weren't improving; they were getting worse. With those prospects, many could choose from three options: limited aspirations, diminished opportunity, or leaving the country.

These early experiences fueled my interest in intellectual property law in the United States, helping to foster creativity for life-saving medicines and scientific advancements. Because my firm was representing the biotechnology industry and pharmaceutical companies, my work required that I study these drugs in some detail. As I delved more into how these drugs worked—how they were created and tested as well as their impact on patient health—I realized that my true vocation was not intellectual property law, even though it was a very honorable profession. My true vocational passion was science and medicine. After mulling over this realization for a few months, I announced to my law firm that I would be leaving soon for medical school. After graduating from medical school several years later, I focused my residency on psychiatry with a particular interest in the neurophysiology of mental health. I furthered my training with two fellowships (medical specialty programs) in pediatric and forensic psychiatry.

With my background in law and medicine, I thought the most obvious career path to pursue would be the field of forensics. During my training and work in forensics, I was often asked by the courts to evaluate a defendant's mental condition, draft a brief for the court, and provide expert testimony. My evaluations often concerned children who were removed from their homes due to an unsafe or untenable family circumstance, or who were on trial for some sort of misdeed or problem they might have caused. Many of these kids suffered from mental health issues; some were prescribed psychiatric and neurological medications and others abused illegal drugs. In certain cases, these adolescents were using illicit substances during the time that they committed some sort of offense. I was sometimes asked if the drugs they were taking created mitigating circumstances that might have an impact on the remedies the courts would mandate, which ranged from undergoing extensive therapy, medication, or substance abuse treatment (if applicable), to performing community service and sometimes spending time in jail. It turned out that this experience in forensics would become the decisive turning point in my career that led me to holistic medicine.

While I was dealing with adolescents in the court system, I wasn't just dealing with some abstract analysis of what kind of medications they were on. I was also often interacting with them and their families on a more personal level. In my conversations with parents, they would often ask me for some general advice concerning the medications their kids were taking. A question that came up over and over was, "What are the potential long-term effects of some of these meds?" This simple question put me in a difficult position. I had a hard time looking them in the eye and giving them a confident answer about long-term effects because, for many of these new medications, we just don't know.

This moral quandary—prescribing health solutions with short-term benefits that might produce more long-term problems—forced me to consider whether there could be a way to improve health outcomes related to Western medical practices, especially concerning medications. After some soul searching, I found that I'm an advocate for change in the form of continuous improvement while keeping an open mind as to how that improvement might take shape. Despite some of the shortcoming of new drugs, overall I am a firm believer in and advocate for Western medicine because it saves lives through cutting-edge medical techniques, devices, and pharmacology. We are fortunate to have it at our disposal when needed. But we can make improvements to our current approach that tends to favor medication as a primary tool used to address mental health issues faced by adolescents.

Some medications that bring about short-term improvements in a person's mental health are quite new; ideally we'd like to have more data on long-term effects. We have to wait for years until people have actually taken a particular medication for a while. In the meantime, people using these psychopharmaceuticals may or may not experience adverse effects over time. So, it dawned on me: While I was a lawyer protecting the creativity that was necessary to develop life-saving drugs, pharmaceutical companies highlighted the short-term, more immediate medication benefits but paid less attention to the long-term consequences that might emerge from taking a particular drug.

Some adolescents and their families that I worked with in the court system and in general clinical practice refused these medications; or, if they were already taking them, they did not want to increase dosages if symptoms decreased but persisted. There had to be a way to give these patients alternatives to conventional medication or possibilities for relief from adverse symptoms arising from those medications.

In looking for other options, I started to think back on two important influences in my life. First, I remembered some important details from my days as an intellectual property lawyer involved in patenting new drugs. In arguing that a drug deserved a patent, I had to provide a very detailed description of what similar things already existed, and how this new medication was developed in a distinctive way. So I got to know these medications pretty well. It turned out that many times the source of a particular medication is something in nature—some chemical compound in a leaf or a root, for instance—that had certain attributes. It could make you sleepy, or reduce pain, for instance. Once scientists isolated that active compound from the plant, it was easy to synthesize it. The important difference between the natural and synthesized versions of these compounds was that the man-made versions were much stronger and purer than those found in nature. This made them act more quickly, but their side effects might be more significant. I considered the plants that formed the foundations of many compounds that I drafted patents for. I surmised that there might be more complex systems within the plants themselves with lots of potential for therapeutic application, not just one compound per plant. A typical plant has literally hundreds of chemical constituents that form its structure and functions. These compounds work synergistically to provide everything from bacterial resistance to regenerative capacity to hormone activity for growth and reproduction.

Second, imagining different plants with their particular healing qualities reminded me of the days when, as a young girl, I spent a lot of time in former

Yugoslavia with my family. Many of my family members used holistic and herbal treatments all the time since many people, especially those living in the countryside and mountainous regions, found it difficult to access more conventional Western medical treatments. For this reason, they often relied on their traditional approaches to healing and wellness. More importantly, the region features lots of natural settings and still maintains many rural and forested areas, traditional agriculture, and native vegetation, where people have easy access to those plants.

I remember my grandmother, Baba, introducing me to a wide range of what we in the United States might now call holistic treatments. In her eyes, she just saw these remedies and palliatives as time-tested methods to help get through the day. Chamomile and lavender grew in parts of southwestern Serbia where my father grew up. Baba would use chamomile for a lot of things, especially an upset stomach. Cinnamon was always abundant in the local markets and used either in tisanes or in meals. (By the way, researchers have found that cinnamon can help people with type 2 diabetes control glucose levels [Magistrelli & Chezem, 2012].) And I often drank a mug of goat's milk with cinnamon before bed rather than cow's milk. It was abundant and considered to be a nutrient-dense healthy substance as well as a good sleep aid. (Today, we know goat's milk has a fair amount of tryptophan, an essential amino acid and precursor to serotonin and melatonin, which are biomolecules that play a role in normal sleep.) (EFSA Panel, 2012) Once in bed, I'd often sleep with some lavender under my pillow. To some, that might sound a bit out of the ordinary or even extravagant for a little girl. But with the flowers blooming in the region and nearby hills, it was easy for my grandmother to give me something to make my night restful and soothing. I felt very well taken care of.

These childhood experiences helped me to quell my own adult consternation in the face of parents who were anxious to know how psychiatric medications were going to affect their children. Following lengthy discussions regarding pharmaceutical treatments and their potential short- and long-term side effects, I felt inspired to set out on a path that, in the long term, would provide safe and viable alternative therapies and complementary options for those concerned with improving mental health: for patients (along with their parents or caregivers) who declined conventional drug therapies as well as for those who wanted synergistic therapies that could complement mainstream treatments for mental health. Having my feet firmly planted in the soil of Western medicine and evidence-based science, I would make sure to test and examine holistic treatments thoroughly before recommending that anybody use them. From this platform, I was determined to find out more.

Now that I was ready to take this next step into exploring integrative and holistic medicine, an opportunity arose for me to learn more: courses on clinical acupuncture offered by Harvard Medical School. It was called Structural Acupuncture for Physicians, a year-long program to become educated and certified in medical acupuncture. I went in the program as a doubting Thomas, but curiosity won over skepticism. How else was I going to know if these approaches really worked unless I tried to see what they were all about? A wonderful group of physicians from the Harvard community taught the course.

As it turned out, I learned a lot from the dedicated and experienced group of physicians who taught this fascinating subject matter. Even more impressive was how much I learned from other students. My fellow students came from a wide array of medical fields: anesthesia, internal medicine, obstetrics and gynecology, sports medicine and rehabilitation, and surgery. I believe I was the only psychiatrist in the year-long course. Our collective experience and points of view improved all of our approaches immensely. That was one of the most eye-opening years that I had in medicine.

I followed this up with a medical acupuncture fellowship at Boston Medical Center in clinical acupuncture, offered by their department of internal medicine. The other certification programs I completed over several years included Chinese herbal medicine, Indian Ayurveda, and regenerative and functional medicine.

From the very beginning of embarking on this journey, I was impressed by one thing: results. In class, students discussed research about the positive impact of integrative and holistic medicine. But even more impressive was what I saw in our weekend and evening clinicals, where we would treat patients who would come on an ad hoc basis. I was amazed by the positive response of these patients to the treatments. I started out seeing patients with relatively small problems, like restricted movement in their shoulders. As time went on, I was exposed to everything from chronic migraines to infertility to palliative care for cancer patients. In all of these cases, to varying degrees, integrative care techniques made a difference. I realized that some portion or degree of their response could be placebo effect. Nonetheless, the overall response to these treatments was significant. All sorts of problems, both physical and psychological complaints, showed improvement.

So, the doubting Thomas in me needed proof, and here it was: a wide range of patients with a host of different problems getting better clinically. And there was no reason for them to report feeling this way, no secondary gain or incentive to report improvement unless it was really happening. To see the relief that these patients experienced made a profound impression on me.

Moreover, many patients who came to see me for conventional psychiatric treatment would ask, without being prompted, about integrative treatments. I could only provide referrals to outside providers or information on other holistic treatment facilities that they could pursue on their own because these treatments had not yet been fully incorporated into current medical practice. This was frustrating because there were so many advantages to integrative medicine:

- These approaches worked. They didn't cure everything, of course, but they had a positive impact on patients' lives.
- They were cost effective, often priced at a small fraction of conventional medical treatments.
- They were versatile, as they could be applied at a variety of times and places.
- They offered options to patients who declined conventional medical treatment for various reasons:
  - Those on current medications who wanted added treatment options but not increased medication dosages.
  - Those on high-dose meds who did not experience full symptom relief and were in search of additional therapies.
- They gave patients a sense of empowerment because they now had the tools to treat themselves effectively whenever they felt the need.
- On a much larger scale, these approaches can become a powerful component in our society's move toward encouraging more preventive health care through:
  - Educating our patient population about their own health needs.
  - Teaching patients to recognize early signs and symptoms of mental health problems.
  - Promoting greater mindfulness about their current conditions.

So it then occurred to me to ask, How could the great potential of these methods be shared with more people? How could integrative health care be transformed from fringe therapies to normal activities—just one more arrow in the quiver of methods available to help people stay healthy? Maybe the easiest way to do this, I thought, might be one that is most familiar to people in Western societies: Subject these therapies to rigorous scientific scrutiny. Sure, word of mouth is powerful testimony, but it cannot be scaled effectively to convince society at large. What I needed was verifiable, publishable data. Later, I would apply all of this broad training in integrative and holistic medicine to the creation and design of a unique program of research that would enable me to gather data about these treatments.

WHEN I SET out to create an evidence-based research program that could evaluate the feasability and efficacy of integrative and holistic methods for improving mental health, I wanted to aim my efforts at a population for whom this could have the most benefit. In my training in psychiatry, I was often struck by how teenagers were particularly vulnerable to mental health issues. Going through so much change, teens are simultaneously growing and learning in marvelous ways, but all that plasticity makes them particularly fragile in the face of stresses and crises they may encounter. Also, many treatments delivered for adolescents are constructed from research on adults. As Frances Jensen shows in her book *The Teenage Brain*, kids' and adults' brains are very different (Jensen & Nutt, 2015). Kids have long been badly served by this eliding of teen and adult physiology into one indistinguishable lump. Conducting a research program focusing specifically on teens would help address this imbalance of available data.

So I designed a treatment protocol that consisted of a series of complementary and alternative medicine therapies, or CAM, which included medical acupuncture, 100% natural plant-based essential oils for aromatherapy, and sound therapy using precise-frequency tuning forks. Within a 30-minute treatment, all three modalities were used for each weekly session. The protocol consisted of eight treatments (once a week). Since this type of study had not been conducted previously, one of the research aims was to utilize several different CAM therapies and throw a broad net to help determine whether any of the treatments were efficacious.

I was fortunate to receive program and research funding that allowed me to bring integrative treatment to adolescents at their high school clinics. This formed the basis of a new school-based program in the Department of Psychiatry at Massachusetts General Hospital: The Integrative Health Program (IHP). I launched the program in collaboration with Chelsea High School just outside of Boston in January 2011. As word of the positive outcomes from Chelsea spread among Boston-area high schools, I received requests from other schools and we soon expanded to Revere and Cambridge. At the same time, I applied for human research approval through the IRB (institutional review board) at my hospital. Once approved, formal study could commence and the data gathered from IRB-approved studies could then be readily published in peer-reviewed medical journals. With my IRB approval, I was now ready both to launch the school-clinic program and to conduct formal research with the IHP participants.

Many of the students in these schools came from low-income households, which meant that they often couldn't afford conventional mental health treatment. And because of logistical difficulties (like parents taking time off from work) and the stigma attached to seeing a "shrink," most low-income kids didn't even think of seeking treatment for their mental health ills. Placing these clinics in schools sometimes felt like getting a spy behind enemy lines. The clinics could sneak behind poverty and prejudice to gain some ground for adolescents in their battles against stress, sleep disorders, fatigue, and other common ailments confronting this segment of the teen population.

Everything we have done in the clinics is designed to maximize ease of access to mental health therapies:

- As we will see in the following chapters, these therapies are very easy for adolescents to administer safely to themselves.
- Each visit to the clinic is only 30 minutes long.
- Thanks to the brevity of the visits, a patient doesn't have to miss much class.
- Because kids like the ease of access combined with the positive results, they end up encouraging their friends to come, which sharply reduces the traditional stigma associated with mental health treatment

These adolescents also came home enthusiastically reporting their progress, thus helping to familiarize their parents with the benefits of these integrative treatments. Suddenly, family members begin to speak more openly about stress and anxiety. When families can find ways to talk about their problems more openly, it has the potential to improve mental health conditions for the communities where they live.

One of the greatest outcomes of these therapies proved to be one of the most surprising—at least for me. It was a sense of empowerment, control, and confidence the kids gained about dealing with their own health. In the past, conventional medicine often found patients as passive receivers of doctors' advice, with little information offered to them about the treatments they were receiving. Times have certainly changed, but conventional medicine is just beginning to understand the great potential of patient empowerment.

When kids come out of a few months of integrative therapies and supportive care through completing the IHP at their respective high school clinics, they often have a clear idea of how they should feel when they are in good health. We have them learn what mental and physical states are healthy and which are not. More importantly, when they find holistic therapies that take them from unhealthy to healthy (e.g., stress to relaxation; sleepiness to alertness), they experience that feeling of wellness and understand on a visceral level what it means to be healthy. They can take the tools (i.e., therapies) and the experience (i.e., moving from feeling unhealthy to healthy) with them the rest of their lives and advocate for their own health needs armed with this knowledge and training. And, with a little luck, they can pass what they've learned on to their friends and even their own children and grandchildren, just like my grandmother did for me when I was young.

Acknowledgments

//

SOME THINGS WE create are best done through collaboration. This book was no exception. I'm extending deep thanks to those whose work was selfless and generous. If it weren't for each of you, the words on the pages that follow would not exist. To all the Boston-area school clinics that had the vision and progressive thought to allow the Integrative Health Program into their schools: Chelsea High School, Revere High School, Cambridge Rindge and Latin High School. At those clinics I met some of the most dedicated clinicians and clinical staff: Jordan Hampton, Anne Berrian, Betty Munson, Teresa Grignon, Wanda Vega and Maria Lapop. As I embarked on this journey of integrative treatments all of your efforts contributed to the most important outcome—the wellness of our patients. I want to express my deepest gratitude to Dr. Nancy Rappaport, who has been a supervisor and mentor during and since my medical fellowship training. And also to: Drs. Mary Lyons-Hunter and Diane Greer whose support at our MGH clinic was critically important. And, to the people who helped me copyedit this book, correct my unintelligible prose, and keep my references in good form—Mark Rennella and Michelle Nicholasen.

Introduction

////////////////////////////////

WHEN CHILDREN COME into this world, their parents usually want the best possible future for them—good schools, good friends, and a safe and secure environment in which they can learn about the world. And, of course, parents want their little ones to be healthy and happy.

But our children face a lot of challenges to maintain happiness and good health as they become teenagers. In fact, the situation can seem pretty bleak for some parents today as they face an unhappy truth: Adolescents in the United States are stressed out, physically tired, and diagnosed with various medical conditions in epidemic proportions. Left badly or inadequately treated, these mental illnesses have a snowball or metastatic effect, just like any other medical condition. As with minor illnesses like bronchitis or high blood pressure, conditions such as low mood, sleep disorders, and stress, to name but a few, worsen and become more pervasive and deeply embedded pathologies when left untreated.

The rates of these pathologies are indeed distressing. Take depression. "The US National Institute of Mental Health (NIMH) and World Health Organization (WHO) estimate that in the US, depression is the leading cause of disability and worldwide it is the 2nd leading contributor to the global burden of disease for persons 15 to 44 years old" (Murray & Lopez, 1996). Symptoms of depression can include loss of positive associations and sense of achievement, negative thoughts, irritability, changes in sleeping patterns, and hopelessness (Ljubi-novic, 2015). For adolescents, depression and anxiety can be devastating and can interfere not only with day-to-day living, but peer relationships, which are so important at that life stage.

The debilitating condition of clinical depression often has symptoms of despair, guilt, exhaustion, pain, and anxiety. Adolescents who suffer from this condition find it hard to become motivated or enthused about any part of life. Rising rates of teen suicide are an alarming warning that depression is out of control and growing rapidly. Current trends show that by 2020 depression will be the second leading cause of disability worldwide, trailing only ischemic heart disease (Murray & Lopez, 1996).

With these troubling trends facing adolescents and their families, wouldn't every parent—and every teacher, counselor, school nurse, and therapist—want every available tool at their disposal to remove the impediments to their children's well-being? Unfortunately, when it comes to dealing with mental health issues facing our young population today, the most well-known and widely used approaches are not enough. Often, they simply amount to being too little, too late to make a major impact on the lives of our children. The intent of this book is to start addressing the insufficiency of current approaches to mental health treatments by offering more tools, more options, and more possibilities to lift the spirits of adolescents with hope for real improvements to their lives. While people of all ages would benefit from additional mental health treatments, I focus on treatments for adolescents ages 13–19.

Many of the tools I suggest in this book are derived from what has been referred to as holistic or alternative medicine. The adjectives describing these types of medical treatments are apt, but they also can carry a stigma among many in the West as being unconventional or unreliable. I'd like to suggest that instead of being just alternative that the treatments I discuss can also be understood as offering (when used in conjunction with conventional medicine) a path to more comprehensive and satisfactory care options for adolescent mental health. We need to do away with believing there is a bright line separating conventional and alternative medicine. In some cases, these different therapeutic approaches have similar origins as well as scientifically proven efficacy.

Understanding their similarities helps us to see these approaches as complementary, not antagonistic. One of my goals is to provide an evidence-based, how-to approach for school clinicians, counselors, teachers, and parents to employ holistic approaches to implementing integrative techniques for common cognitive and behavioral conditions experienced by adolescents. And the most exciting element about these tools of alternative medicine is that many of them are easy for kids to learn and apply by themselves. What could be more reassuring to a parent than knowing that their kids are becoming self-sufficient?

The new health care that is emerging today embraces both conventional and complementary therapies. While some may perceive a wide gulf between these two kinds of therapies, scholars of the history of medicine have long understood that medicine has combined many different approaches for centuries. Steven M. Oberhelman explains that anthropologists have found an interesting commonality in most health care systems across time:

> In a society, there exists not a single medical system, but multiple systems. Individuals resort to one or another of these systems for a variety of reasons, such as economic means, accessibility of medical practitioners, the form of illness, the healer's past success or his reputation for dealing with specific ailments, and the previous experiences of the patient and her family and friends. (2013, p1.)

Although every era has its good and bad medical practices, its therapeutic breakthroughs as well as its quackery, the lines that separate these two camps are not strictly determined by the discipline of medical practice used to treat any specific ailment or its symptoms.

The scholarship on medical practices in ancient Greece is especially revealing. The history of Greek medicine is important because Greece is the birthplace of Hippocrates (460–370 B.C.), arguably the father of modern scientific Western medical practice and the originator of the Hippocratic oath.* Yet at the same time Hippocrates was gaining fame and stature, the sick and ailing

---

*One of the most famous passages in the oath is, "With regard to healing the sick, I will devise and order for them the best diet, according to my judgment and means; and I will take care that they suffer no hurt or damage."

in ancient Greece could and did consult a wide variety of healers: the gods (through temple medicine), magicians, midwives, root cutters (who collected medically beneficial plants and sold them at markets), drug sellers, botanists, gymnastic trainers, and dieticians. The more scientifically inclined of these healers—those who followed the Hippocratic school of medicine—did not earn respect in society through a diploma or advanced degree. Instead, they competed in the wide free market of ideas and practices that were available to everyone. The reputation of doctors "ultimately rested on [their] successes and failures" (Oberhelman, 2013).

How a patient might use the medical resources available to him in this marketplace could vary greatly. For example, as Oberhelman points out, a sick person might consult both a physician and a priest, "especially if the source of illness [was] seen by the patient in supernatural terms." Conversely, and less obviously, the basis of much rational medicine could be found in many more traditional practices:

> These various medical practitioners often overlapped in theory and [practice]. In the healing cult of the god Asclepius, sick patients would come and sleep at night in a sleeping chamber. The god visited the sick person and healed by direct intervention . . . or indirectly by sending a dream in which he recommended a treatment. The instructions in the dream were often straight out of Hippocratic medicine: bloodletting, baths, diet, exercise, drugs, poultices, emetics, and the like. Hippocratic writers, on their part, possessed a religious outlook; they invoked the gods and called on their patronage, and recommended prayers as a useful companion to medical treatment. (Oberhelman, 2013, p. 9)

The intimate connections between traditional and modern medicine might also be exemplified in modern drugs. The active ingredient in aspirin, for example, is a form of salicin, a compound derived from plants. The Greeks, Hippocrates among them, counseled using salicin in a drink that could mollify labor pains. As in most medicines, the modern equivalent of salicin used in aspirin, acetylsalicylic acid, is much purer and stronger than salicin and has a more direct impact on the body. It also has more side effects. The more ancient form of aspirin worked more slowly, but had a more mild and gradual impact on the patient. As one might imagine, some forms of aspirin are better than others, depending on the patient's needs.

Examples from the roots of modern medical practice are highly instructive because they point out that pluralism has long been embedded in Western medical practices, whether acknowledged or not. What we should learn from this is that many (not all, of course, but many) more traditional or what we often refer to as holistic medical practices have been the starting point of Western medical therapies. Moreover, modern medicine is beginning to discover the role of the mental dispositions of patients (e.g., levels of stress, happiness, depression) in responding well to conventional treatments. These dispositions also have real long-term impact on physical health.

By encouraging the crucial role of patients in their own healing, many more health care providers are trying to promote various methods of self-healing. Because many of the drugs and therapies used by modern medicine have pre-modern forms that are still easy for people to access and apply to themselves, providers from all over the health care spectrum are encouraging their patients to work with these older therapies. That is one reason why today's health care system (conventional and holistic) is so much more patient-centered than even 20 or 30 years ago. We're coming full circle; now, medical practices are being judged mostly by results, not only by medical credentials. And those results are improved through patient empowerment in their own recoveries from illness as well as in the continual maintenance of their own well-being.

Throughout this book, you will be introduced to a variety of integrative techniques that have proven useful to adolescents, and scenarios illustrating how the patients applied them in their daily lives. As background and context, I include an explanation of what is known about the medical and physiological underpinnings of a particular disorder, such as chronic headaches or sleep disturbances. But the medical explanation does not give a complete picture. When we look at a patient as a whole person, the interconnection between body and emotions becomes clearer. For adolescents, and indeed for all of us, stresses and problems reside in the physical, emotional, and developmental realms. The integrative approach to helping teens incorporates all spheres of concern. Most important, it reinforces teenagers' need for independence by giving them the tools to self-administer. Ultimately it teaches them that feeling better is truly within their control.

Whether you are a medical practitioner, counselor, or parent, in the following pages you will find evidence for viable and valid forms of intervention that can be added, without risk, to your knowledge base for helping to heal the adolescents in your life, and in your practice. It's an exciting new way of looking at mental health: teaching teens how to help themselves, not just for the challenges of the moment, but as a lifelong skill.

HOLISTIC HEALTH
for ADOLESCENTS

CHAPTER 1

A Critical Role:
Adolescent Integrative Medicine

//

TODAY'S INTEGRATIVE MEDICINE addresses the mind, body, and spiritual aspects of health and seeks to rebuild a bridge between conventional and alternative medical systems (Maizes, Rakel, & Niemiec, 2009). The integrative approach to treatment is especially important to adolescents who are undergoing rapid change, which includes increasing social pressures, mounting responsibility, and uncertain self-identity. Behavioral and emotional problems are not uncommon during this period of the life span, and educating adolescents about the sensory aspects of their bodies can help them to learn self-regulation.

A multisensory therapeutic approach is an effective and efficient way to help adolescents reach this goal of self-regulation. The treatment protocols described in this book are therefore organized in a multisensory structure. Each ailment is treated by engaging the five senses: touch, sight, smell, sound, and taste. A particular sense-specific holistic modality (e.g., acupressure for sense of touch, clinical aromatherapy essential oils for sense of smell) is used to stimulate a sensory pathway and induce positive change and healing. This form of treatment is the basis for full-stimuli immersion of the senses for various mental health conditions.

In other words, the mental health tools for adolescents I describe in this book are applied to (and through) the senses. Using the senses as the pathway to mental therapy has three distinct advantages: (1) The senses are foundational not just to our well-being, but also to our being, our sense of self; (2) sensory stimuli affect us every day—we need to learn how to channel these stimuli to make us feel better, not worse; and (3) the senses are easy to access, requiring little or no technological gadgets or highly skilled expertise to leverage.

As the brain takes in sensory stimuli through its receptors (the eyes, skin, nose, etc.), these stimuli can arouse the activity of wide-reaching components of the brain's networks. From a neurological standpoint, as we interact and engage in daily activities, our bodies are continuously inundated with stimuli. The integration of these stimuli and our brain's interpretation of this information is what allows our bodies to react and respond to the environment. The importance of the senses becomes clearer when we understand that they were and continue to be absolutely essential for day-to-day survival. To be useful for survival, the brain needs to make sense of sensory inputs. It does this by interpreting these sensory messages as, on one hand, something positive, soothing, or healing, or, on the other hand, something harmful, painful, or noxious (Chudler, 2015).

This is why the senses have such an important impact on our moods. The tight connection of senses to emotions could be seen as a very successful evolutionary adaptation to our environment. Imagine the usefulness of this connection in the days when early humans had few technological advantages over the animals that threatened them. If a human sensed (through smell, sight, hearing) that there was danger close by in the form of some threatening animal like a lion or a bear, feeling fear became a tool of survival, and perhaps decisively quickened his reaction (along with his step), so he could live another day. "Based on a study of 190-million-year-old fossils, paleontologist Tim Rowe of the University of Texas has proposed that the reason that mammals (including humans) have larger, more complex brains than other animals is that mammals needed a larger brain to improve their sense of smell—and thus their chances of survival" (National Geographic Channel, 2011).

As technology has created a buffer between humans and animals that could threaten us on a daily basis, the fight-or-flight reaction to danger has, perhaps, become less useful. But because the connection between our senses and our state of being is so fundamental, we humans are still hard-wired to respond to our environment in a very sensitive and comprehensive manner. But instead of listening for the rustle of grass in the quiet savannah or smelling for the scent of silent predator or prey, modern humans are often surrounded by the whirring sights of the city or the bells and whistles of technological devices. In fact, we often deliberately connect these devices directly to our senses (e.g., earbuds). Even if we find these sensory inputs pleasing, the rate, variety, and sheer volume of this input is exponentially greater than it ever was for our ancestors. It's difficult for the primitive foundations of our brains to cope with all this external activity. Our response to sensory inputs comes in the form of a physiological reaction. This can include the release of neurotransmitters in the brain, a cascade of hormones, and inflammatory reactions, to name a few.

Luckily, humans can adapt to new, modern circumstances in two ways. First, the level of neurological activity in response to external signaling is adaptable and flexible. Second, to a great degree, the kind of sensory stimuli we receive can be similarly flexible. In other words, we can actually often choose what kind of sensory stimuli our brains have to interpret and, in the process, help to rewire or recondition our brains to create a healthier sensory environment. Modern science has recently confirmed certain truths that some ancient healers understood intuitively: that the brain can adapt and change to new circumstances, a condition described in the modern medical profession as neuroplasticity. Neuroplasticity allows us to reteach the brain and the senses to which it is connected to return to their natural equilibrium—which lets our bodies do what they need to do to create a foundation for happiness.

Our bodies possess a powerful innate capacity to promote healing when provided with the appropriate intervention. Stimulating our sensory pathways with positive signals can influence our response to pain, immunity, the stress response, circadian rhythms, and illness. Knowing this, a logical approach to calming the excited or depressed adolescent brain is to find a path through the senses that can influence the brain in a positive way. One powerful remedy is to provide a wide-ranging platform—a guided menu of approaches—that would introduce positive holistic therapies in the form of multisensory stimuli. This platform would then prime the brain to support reactions of decreased pain, increased relaxation, and healing.

The platform could be effective in both short-term and long-term therapeutic programs. In the short term, it can reduce and help suppress some of the most acute symptoms of bad mental states. In the long term, used repeatedly

over time, these programs have an additive effect that can have more permanent impact.

While this sensory platform might seem new, in reality it incorporates individual therapeutic elements that have been used for centuries by some indigenous
peoples, ethnic groups, and various cultures around the globe. The application
of the multisensory approach combined with modern scientific analysis forms
the basis for cutting-edge application of these techniques. This type of evaluation heightens the clinical relevance and use of these remedies.

Of course, the science and research behind these therapies require careful
consideration. In the vast field of integrative treatment, not all modalities possess the same degree of rigorous testing. Any informed decision to utilize holistic
techniques requires an extensive review of the current medical literature. This
allows us to provide our patients and users the best opportunity for symptom
relief and healing. Some of the sensory treatments and tools we'll be reviewing
include: acupuncture and acupressure, clinical aromatherapy, yoga and meditation, sound and music therapy, and herbal and tea remedies. And in the chapters
that follow, I refer to medical literature to help explain the physiological mechanisms that are leveraged through these treatments.

AS MENTIONED ABOVE, this book offers options to help to heal a wide variety of mental health problems faced by adolescents by using therapies closely
aligned with the senses as a primary vehicle of treatment. But before we get
to the problems and the nuances of their specific treatments, it will be useful
first to introduce readers to the importance of the individual senses in human
development along with the complementary therapy most closely aligned with
a particular sense.

In some respects, telling readers that they will receive an introduction to
the importance of the senses seems almost preposterous because the senses
are what introduce every human to the world. Their impact on our personalities
and well-being cannot be underestimated, but because they are so basic and
integral to our being and survival that we tend to take them for granted. (If our
personalities and well-being could be compared to the colors of a painting, the
senses are the oil and pigment that make those colors possible.) Additionally, in
our modern circumstances often characterized by speed and massive amounts

of stimulation, taking the time to appreciate the wonderfully complex and subtle nuances of our sensory inputs can be difficult.

To understand the power of the senses, we do have to slow down and examine them one by one. As you will understand by the end of this book, each individual sense has its own specific and significant portal to our health and well-being. Knowing what each individual sense can do helps to explain why these complementary therapies can act so powerfully upon us. Moreover, after appreciating how one sense works upon us, it becomes clear how using multiple senses in combination within therapeutic contexts can potentially multiply their power exponentially.

An important fact about the human senses that makes them unique comes into focus when we understand that, despite their importance to human development, they are often unimpressive compared to the sensory array employed by animals. Not only are animal sense receptors often much more powerful than those of humans (a bloodhound's nose, for instance), but they also often have different senses than we do. Take, for instance, bats that use their own kind of radar to create aural maps of their surroundings in a split second, allowing them to avoid obstacles or track down prey in midair.

The thing that distinguishes the human senses from those of most animals is that they are backed by the huge computing power of the human brain (Shreeve, 2015). This complicated intimacy between brains and senses sometimes does not encourage the best approach to survival. When we quickly and reflexively remove our hands from a source of heat, for example, we deploy our motor (involuntary) reflexes to pull away from danger. But, more often than not, our brains and our senses work very closely together in ways that make the separation between one (a sense) and the other (the brain) difficult to determine.

Take our sense of sight, for instance. Physiologically, as we will discuss later in more detail, the retina, which is often described as part of the eye, is actually part of the brain. And despite the huge amount of neurological power devoted to seeing—which dwarfs that of any other sense—the brain still must compensate for what the eye can't see. This happens in the case of the brain filling in the incomplete picture of the world delivered by the eye—a picture that is incomplete because of permanent blind spots that the eye has naturally (Grady, 1993; for a very accessible overview of recent vision research, see Hagen, 2012). Vision, in other words, does not simply create a neurological record of the objective world. It is, in some ways, subjective—or subjectively constructed for the benefit of survival. In the words of one researcher, "We learn to see" (David Knill, quoted in Hagen, 2012).

In this chapter, we'll examine the senses in this order:

Hearing

Taste

Smell

Touch

Sight*

HEARING: SOUND AND MUSIC THERAPIES

The Sense of Hearing

For humans, processing sound happens on a 24-hour basis from birth. We know this because scientists have recorded how the brain processes sound during sleep. For infants, that 24/7 exposure to sound stimulates, develops, and shapes important neural networks in the brain, especially those for spoken and written language. What's more, for the purposes of music therapy, the brain is hard-wired to respond to music and rhythms. Parents of hearing-impaired children are encouraged to sing while communicating.

The sense of hearing develops throughout the brain. If, hypothetically, a child was deprived of sound for a year, the entire brain would continue to develop without sound as an input, thus changing the (normal) development of the entire brain. One professional in this field recommends that families with deaf or hearing-impaired children get hearing aids or implants that the children should wear continuously to ensure "auditory brain development." She explains:

We know that if the desired outcome is spoken communication and literacy, then hearing, and by hearing we mean auditory brain development,

*Sight takes up a huge amount of neuronal hardware, more than any other human sense (National Geographic TV, 2015).

is a first-order event. Obviously, there is not one little nugget in the brain that has *auditory* written on it; auditory tissue is located *throughout* the brain. All of those areas need stimulation in order to develop, and they cannot be stimulated if there is a hearing loss unless we have technology that gets sound to the brain. (Flexer, 2011)

Left undeveloped, the parts of the brain that are normally set aside for processing sound can be co-opted by other senses, especially the sense of sight (Flexer, 2011; see also Biranholz & Benacerraf, 1983). This may be the dark side of neuroplasticity: If you don't use a sense, you can lose it.

There are, broadly speaking, three stages of development of the human auditory system. In the first phase, during the second trimester of pregnancy, a fetus's cochlea (which is the auditory version of the inner ear) reaches "virtual full maturation." A fetus then begins responding to sound during the late third trimester of pregnancy. In the second phase, which occurs during the perinatal period (spanning the few weeks before and after birth), brain stem structures related to hearing undergo rapid development. The third phase of development is unusually long, compared to the other senses. The cortex development related to hearing (located in the brain's temporal lobes) takes about a decade, as opposed to approximately a year for the other senses. This long maturation time reflects both the "anatomical complexity [of the auditory cortex] and its role in the multiyear process of language acquisition" (Moore & Linthicum, 2007; see also Biranholz & Benacerraf, 1983).

Sound Therapy

Sound therapy has been used for centuries by many cultural, religious, and indigenous groups around the globe: from ancient Greek and Egyptian civilizations, to Vedic Indian culture, to Tibetan chants and mantras, to Aboriginal groups in Australia, and to American native tribes. In the case of ancient Greece, for example, the understanding of the healing potential of music was made clear in how the Greeks integrated music into the description of their gods. Apollo was a god not only associated with the sun, as many may remember him, but also the god of music (Antrim, 1944; see also Cook, 1997; Gaynor, 2002).

The broad category of sound therapy encompasses a wide range of practices. The most prominent form of sound therapy practiced in the United States has been music therapy. Fundamentally, music is organized sound and is a form of treatment well known in conventional medicine. Since the National Association of Music in Hospitals was created in 1926, many hospitals and clinics throughout the United States have developed music therapy programs to benefit and support patient recovery (Edwards, 2007).

Early music therapy programs grew slowly. But rapid growth occurred after World War II when soldiers returned home from the battlefields with emotional and psychological problems. Music and soothing sounds provided relief and played a supportive role in healing. Then, in 1945, the U.S. War Department issued Technical Bulletin 187, which detailed a music therapy program created by the Office of the Surgeon General (American Music Therapy Association, 2014). Music therapy was described as being supportive of occupational therapy and physical reconditioning. As a result of this acceptance by the War Department, music therapy programs grew in hospitals.

Sound and music are noninvasive, simple, and cost-effective therapeutic tools. This form of treatment has been shown to reduce pain and anxiety for children undergoing medical or dental procedures. In addition, when music therapy is combined with other modalities, it may be more effective than when presented alone (Beckhuis, 2009). Sound and music have also been shown to reduce arousal during stress and support a state of calm (Pelletier, 2004). Further, a report by the Cochrane Collaboration, a nonprofit organization evaluating therapies according to the principles of evidence-based medicine, highlighted the physiological effects of this modality and found that music may reduce the effects of coronary artery disease and also decrease blood pressure, heart rate, and respiratory rate (Bradt, Dileo, & Potvin, 2009).

American adolescents listen to approximately 4.5 hours of music per day. The use of sound and music are processes with which they are familiar and which they find easy to adopt (Campbell, Connell, & Beegle, 2007). Some studies have shown that music improves the mood of adolescents by reducing stress and lowering anxiety levels, thereby reducing depression, which is prevalent among adolescents today (Misic, Arandjelovic, Stanojkovic, Vladejic, & Mladenovic, 2010).

The IHP that I founded at Massachusetts General Hospital introduced tuning forks for sound therapy. Tuning forks are U-shaped steel tines that act as acoustic resonators. Once activated, by firmly tapping them on a rubber mallet base, they produce a specific and constant musical pitch that endures for several minutes.

The particular tuning forks used for the IHP were set to emit a pure musical tone at a frequency of 136.1 Hz. There are hundreds of tuning forks of various lengths and mass, each of which produces different, precise sound frequencies. Often they are used to tune musical instruments and are frequently applied in Indian temple music. The IHP chose the 136.1 Hz frequency due to its deeply resonant sound and long-term application in integrative treatments to reduce stress, relieve body tension, and assist in meditative practices.

TASTE: HERBS AND TEAS

The Sense of Taste

The sense of taste is closely related to food intake. Researchers have noted that humans often do not consume food simply to maintain good health and enough energy to function through the day—what might be referred as being in a homeostatic state. But, as we all have experienced, eating food also has a strong correlation with desire and pleasure in humans, thus also making it a hedonic experience. For maintaining a homeostatic state, an individual's decisions concerning the desirability of food can be made without any need to learn culturally or experientially. Humans can (and will) accept or reject a previously unknown food on the basis of taste alone, thus making it a primary (an unlearned) reinforcement of eating behavior.

The behavior exhibited in eating more than we need—for instance, in deciding to get a second big slice of cherry cheesecake after dinner—takes humans well past their necessary calorie intake and into behavior that is hedonic, or eating for pleasure. This is a secondary reinforcement, meaning that it is related to the reward value of certain kinds of taste.

Taste, then, sometimes acts like a reflex (primary reinforcement) and in other instances like a learned behavior (secondary reinforcement). This, of course, means that the impact of taste on the brain is often mixed with many other neural inputs associated with food, such as emotions. It's also mixed with visual, olfactory, and tactile senses that work with taste to determine whether or not a food should be ingested. Although it is sometimes described as one of the weaker senses, it is, nonetheless, a "potent motivational force" (Kringelbach, 2004).

Nutritionists have been keenly interested in studying the sense of taste through infancy and childhood in order to learn how to better steer children toward a varied diet of healthy foods. It is widely accepted today that children "live in different chemical sensory worlds than adults" (Liem & Mennella, 2003). As early as 1877, Charles Darwin noted:

> I will add that formerly it looked to me as if the sense of taste at least with my own children when they were still very young, was different from the adult sense of taste: this shows itself by the fact that they did not refuse rhubarb with some sugar and milk which is for us an abominable disgusting mixture and by the fact that they strongly preferred the most sour and tart fruits, as for instance unripe gooseberries and Holz apples. (quoted in Liem & Mennella, 2003, p. 1)

The reasons behind these sometimes stark differences between adults and children are not exactly clear. Researchers have speculated that some children's preference for sour taste (about 33% of 5- to 9-year-olds compared to 0% in adults in one study) may reflect a parallel interest in thrill seeking and adventure. Or it may just be a natural, unlearned behavior reflecting some maturation process in the palette. Or it could be learned through exposure to certain foods as an infant. Whatever the fundamental reasons behind taste preferences in young children, it is important to remember that these varied preferences and experiences of children often shape the experience of the adolescent and adult, and that these preferences can also vary quite a bit (Liem & Mennella, 2003).

Taste Therapy

"What sustains us, also makes us feel alive," says Paul Freedman (2007) in his book *Food: The History of Taste*. This is certainly true, and what better example than a hot cup of tea late in the afternoon to provide that refreshing, taste-satisfying burst of energy we crave, or that first cup of hot green or black tea in the morning that offers that jolt of caffeine to begin the day. But tea is also a cost-effective, taste-satisfying, stress relief.

Two natural compounds that have been shown to reduce stress levels are found in green and some black teas: (1) L-theanine, one of the predominant amino acids found almost exclusively in tea and historically used as a relaxing agent, has been found to soothe anxiety, without side effects (Lu et al., 2004); (2) catechins, flavonoid phytochemical compounds found principally in green tea and to some extent in black tea, are considered to show the benefits of teas on the biological effects of stress.

Herbal teas are not technically "teas," but tisanes, which are infusions made from plants and herbs. (A true "tea" is made from a variety of the *Camellia sinensis* plant.) A number of herbal tisanes are associated with calming the mind and body and are caffeine-free alternatives to tea. For instance, one writer in the *International Journal of Childbirth Education* recommends chamomile tea for its relaxing properties during a woman's labor and lemon balm or peppermint tea to reduce nausea (Walls, 2009). In our clinic, for example, some of our clients who have been diagnosed with attention-deficit/hyperactivity disorder (ADHD) have found that taking the time out to drink tea during the day has a calming effect.

SMELL: CLINICAL AROMATHERAPY

The Sense of Smell

The sense of smell (or olfaction) plays a somewhat paradoxical role in the human brain. On one hand, smell is not a very precise sense. Humans are often not able to identify smells very reliably, tending instead to point to a range of possibilities ("It smells something like . . ."). This might be explained by the fact that although all information from the nose goes to the olfactory bulb, which is shaped like a thin prong at the front of the brain, where it goes from there varies greatly. That is because the smells often interact with the limbic structures in the brain, which are closely linked to emotions. One researcher of human olfaction writes that "limbic tissue is rather undifferentiated and has rich reciprocal connections between its different structures" (Savic, 2002, p 204). And there's an additional nuance to the perception of smell in the brain, since, "in addition to the input at the olfactory tract, the [olfactory] bulb also receive[s] input from other brain centers that modify . . . neuronal activity" (Strous & Shoenfeld, 2006, p 55).

The inputs received by the nose are also complicated. Humans are able to sense (but perhaps not clearly distinguish between) three different kinds of olfactory input in our "perceptive spectrum": a pure smell (like the whiff of vanilla extract); a combination of smell and input from the trigeminal nerve (which transmits sensations from the face); and pheromones (chemicals emitted from human bodily fluids) (Savic, 2002).

Despite the dispersed impact of olfactory input, the sense of smell may be one of our most primitive and, therefore, most powerfully influential senses on the human being. In 2011, a paleontologist studying ancient mammals used very modern technology (in this case, a computed tomography or CT scan) to theorize that mammals probably evolved bigger brains in order to improve the sense of smell (University of Texas at Austin, 2011). In addition, the interaction of olfactory input with the limbic structure in the brain gives olfaction a pathway to our strong feelings through an "immediate association to emotion and episodic memory" (Savic, 2002).

While the sense of sight (discussed below) certainly uses the most neural hardware of the human senses, some scientists contend that the olfactory system is grossly underrated in the human sensory hierarchy. While it's often pointed out that, for instance, dogs have far more olfactory sensor sells (230 million) than do humans (10 million), "It is suspected . . . that our superior cognitive power allows us to better use olfactory input compared with other mammals" (Hohl, Atzmueller, Fink, & Grammer, 2001). Moreover, olfaction, in the intake of and response to pheromones, plays a very central role in human reproductive behavior. Although it is true that large secretions of pheromones can produce a distinguishable odor, more often than not pheromones are not consciously perceived by humans. Nonetheless, they can often have a powerful connection to our emotions and sexual arousal, "whether or not a chemical stimulus is consciously perceived" (Hohl et al., 2001). So humans often do react to olfactory input without cognitive processing. In other words, the pheromones are particularly important (and, by extension, the importance of the olfactory system in shaping human actions) because they trigger deeply instinctive behavior in all of us (Schall, 1988).

Smell Therapy: Aromatherapy

The use of essential oils for healing has been evident for nearly 6,000 years. The Chinese, Indians, Egyptians, Greeks, and Romans have always used them in cosmetics, perfumes, and drugs. The oils were also used for spiritual, therapeutic, hygienic, and ritualistic purposes. Whether inhaled or applied on the skin, the use of essential oils has become an alternative treatment for infections, stress, and other health problems (Perry & Perry, 2006; for analysis of the impact of aromas on the nervous system of rats, see Wu et al., 2012).

In 1928, René-Maurice Gattefossé, a French chemist, realized the healing properties of lavender oil when he applied it to a burn on his hand that was caused by an explosion in his laboratory. He then applied this discovery to treat burns, skin infections, gangrene, and wounds in soldiers during World War I, and founded the science of aromatherapy. And during World War II, a French army surgeon named Jean Valnet revived the practice (Welsh, 1997). After World War II, Valnet continued to promote aromatherapy and might be considered one of the founders of contemporary approaches to aromatherapy with the publication of his book, *The Practice of Aromatherapy*, published in English in a paperback edition in 1982.

Aromatherapy promotes a sense of relaxation and improves mood. Essential oils such as lavender, rose, orange, bergamot, lemon, and sandalwood have been shown to relieve anxiety, stress, and depression (Herz, 2009). For my teenage clients, I infuse oil into strips of gauze that are stored in a small plastic bag. They can carry the strips and use as needed. At night, spraying lavender on a pillowcase or bed sheets is an effective way to disperse the scent during the wind-down time before bed.

Modern scientific research has also found that the olfactory systems are quite intimately connected to the body's immune systems and can act as a corporeal canary in a coalmine by manifesting some of the earliest symptoms of neurological disorders. For example, "the predictive utility of olfactory identification deficits in patients with mild cognitive impairment has been assessed for follow-up diagnosis of probable Alzheimer's disease." Taking this process a next logical step further, one researcher maintains that

it may be suggested that olfaction may come to play a role in the management and alleviation of various disorders. . . . One interesting illustration of the potential of this paradigm being used in the management of illness is that of the use of fragrance in the treatment of depression and its associated effects on immune function. More specifically, citrus (lemon) fragrance has been shown to restore stress-induced immuno-suppression in rodent models. . . . Remarkably . . . doses of antidepressant medication necessary for the treatment of depression could be markedly reduced following augmentation with citrus fragrance. (Strous & Shoen-feld, 2006, p. 59)

Massage therapy using essential oils often benefits people with depression through the relaxation caused by the combination of scents and massage (Kuri-yama, 2005). As this approach to massage therapy implies, many allopathic therapeutic methods attempt to appeal to more than one sense, either simulta-neously or in succession. While using multiple senses allows therapists greater possibilities of creating benefits for their patients, the procedures for these mul-tisensory treatments are usually both easy to apply and inexpensive.

TOUCH: ACUPUNCTURE AND ACUPRESSURE

The Sense of Touch

Touching is complicated; or one might say that what we understand as touch is more complicated than we often think. It can range from a squeeze of another person's hand to a pat on the head, playing footsie underneath a table, or (less pleasantly) a forceful grab or push. But, as researchers have found, what we sense as touch is deeper than merely making contact with the skin. Touch is part of a tactile means of understanding our environment that includes other outside influences upon the skin, such as temperature, pressure, outside vibra-tions, and how much the skin has to move or stretch in response to coming in contact with another object. The position of one's body through and in relation to one's immediate surrounding space is another job associated with the skin. These complicated processes take place in what is known as the somatosensory system.

For the purposes of adolescent mental health therapy, this book generally uses the word "touch" in its less complicated and more colloquial understanding. But it's important to learn about the complex systems in which touch resides to point out the challenges neurologists face in attempting to describe the exact interaction between touch and the brain. Like the olfactory system, touch deals with many inputs and is also processed in complex neurological pathways. The area in the brain that focuses on touch is on the crown of the head and is called the primary somatosensory cortex, often referred to as S1. But there is also a secondary somatosensory cortex, called S2. Research has confirmed that when human skin is stimulated with painful or nonpainful touch, the S1 and S2 areas both process the stimulus. Why two areas would process one stimulus is uncertain. In fact, researchers are still debating whether or not nonpainful signals for higher primates, such as humans, follow a hierarchical neurological path, going from S1 before going to S2, or if they are processed in both areas at the same time (Lian, Moruraux, & Iannetti, 2011; see also Nelson, Sur, & Kaas, 1980).

The complexity of touch may be attributed to the fact that it could be described as being the first sense of human beings. As one researcher has pointed out, "Long before it has developed ears and eyes and is no more than an inch in length, the human embryo will actively respond to any stimulation of its skin" (Montagu, 1984). With neurological pathways set so deeply, the sense of touch may, in consequence, be very difficult to see clearly and understand precisely.

These deep connections between touch and human development can be more vividly seen in its symptoms—in how touch (or lack of it) impacts the young and adult human. For instance, while frequent and close interactions between infants and their mothers is of undeniable benefit, research on orphaned infants in Europe "suggests the possibility that these orphaned infants are not suffering from maternal deprivation, per se, but from sensory deprivation, and more specifically, a deprivation of mechanosensory stimulation" (Ardiel, 2010). Later in life, both monkeys and human children who lack adequate stimulation through touch often express above-average levels of aggression and violent tendencies (Field, 2002). And the foundational depth of touch in human development may explain its power and importance in communicating feelings that go beyond words. Researchers have found that humans "have an innate ability to decode emotions via touch alone." This ability to communicate in an unspoken (and universal) language is supremely useful in conveying extreme emotions such as "intense grief or fear, but also in ecstatic moments of joy or love—when only the language of touch can fully express what we feel" (Chollot, 2013).

Touch Therapy: Acupuncture

Traditional Chinese medicine (TCM) and other Asian healing practices include acupuncture, which dates back millennia. Based on a review of data, acupuncture is a safe CAM modality for pediatric patients (Jindal, Ge, & Mansky, 2008).

Despite the use of acupuncture for thousands of years in Asia, its acceptance in Western medicine did not gain momentum until the 1980s and beyond. TCM practices slowly made their way from East to West in the 1850s through medical missionaries from England (Ulett, Han, & Han, 1998). As these groups exchanged information, missionaries translated Chinese texts into English.

Acupuncture first gained some significant notice in the United States as a very unexpected outcome of Richard Nixon's famous trip to China in 1972. In late July 1971, James Reston, a reporter for the *New York Times*, was traveling across China to report on the thawing of U.S.-China diplomatic relations. During his visit, Reston underwent an emergency appendectomy using conventional anesthesia in the Anti-Imperialist Hospital in Beijing (Kaplan, 1997). During recovery, he experienced extreme pain that was treated by an acupuncturist, Prof. Li Chang Yuan. In an article about his acupuncture experience, "Now, about My Operation in Peking," Reston described the acupuncture as wholly foreign to his experience, but effective. (Notice his tone as a not-quite-reformed skeptic who had begun to appreciate the apparent potential of acupuncture.) This is how Reston (1971) recalled the experience:

> [Dr. Li] inserted three long, thin needles into the outer part of my right elbow and below my knees and manipulated them in order to stimulate the intestine and relieve the pressure and distension of the stomach.
>
> That sent ripples of pain racing through my limbs and, at least, had the effect of diverting my attention from the distress in my stomach. Meanwhile, Doctor Li lit two pieces of an herb called ai, which looked like the burning stumps of a broken cheap cigar, and held them close to my abdomen while occasionally twirling the needles into action.
>
> All this took about 20 minutes, during which I remember thinking that

it was rather a complicated way to get rid of gas on the stomach, but there was a noticeable relaxation of the pressure and distension within an hour with no recurrence of the problem thereafter.

Being the reporter he was, Reston investigated the background of China's use of acupuncture in hospitals in the 1970s. The main reason he found was the fact that China's peasants, which at the time comprised 80% of China's population, simply could neither access nor afford conventional medical treatments. Acupuncture and other types of TCM, on the other hand, proved to be inexpensive and oftentimes effective at treating many illnesses and conditions. In fact, because of the Cultural Revolution, Dr. Li himself had begun acupuncture training with as much skepticism as Mr. Reston. While Li "had not been a believer in the use of acupuncture techniques," he had to admit that "'a fact is a fact—there are many things they can do'" (Reston, 1971).

Interestingly, Reston jokingly attributed his physical ailments to his psychological distress at having missed the scoop about Henry Kissinger's secret trip to China in early July. "Without a single shred of supporting medical evidence, I trace my attack of acute appendicitis to Henry A. Kissinger of the White House staff. He arrived in China on July 9. My wife and I arrived in South China the day before." Right after learning that he had missed the scoop that Kissinger had been in Peking [Beijing] to plan a meeting between Nixon and Mao the next year, Reston writes, "At that precise moment, or so it seems, the first stab of pain went through my groin. By evening I had a temperature of 103, and in my delirium I could see Mr. Kissinger floating across my bedroom ceiling grinning at me out of the corner of a hooded rickshaw." Reston's story and the picture that accompanied it created a short flurry of interest by medical doctors in the United States. Although initial investigations into acupuncture following Reston's article tended to be inconclusive in the United States, Reston's report made the practice much more familiar to Americans than it had ever been before.

Western medicine has made numerous attempts to explain acupuncture's mechanism of action from an allopathic perspective. While it has yet to be fully elucidated, certain aspects have gained general acceptance. First, many of the over 350 acupuncture points correspond to nerve bundles or muscle trigger points. Neuroimaging studies show that acupuncture can calm areas of the brain that register pain and activate those involved in downregulating the stress response (Dhond, Kettner, & Napadow, 2007). Doppler ultrasound has shown that acupuncture increases blood flow in treated areas (Lo, Lin, Ong, & Sun, 2013; see also Stux, Berman, & Pomeranz, 2000). Finally, thermal imaging shows that acupuncture can decrease inflammation (Santos et al., 2013).

Another study conducted an extensive literature review to evaluate the role of acupuncture in anxiety conditions. Results showed statistically significant effects directly attributable to acupuncture treatment. It should be noted that the author discussed the need for improved study design, to lend influence and support to the use of acupuncture to significantly reduce the symptoms of anxiety disorders (Errington-Evans, 2011). Similar studies about acupressure—a similar practice that applies pressure to certain parts of the body but without needles—report its promising use in alleviating symptoms of many ailments ranging from fatigue to nausea in cancer patients undergoing treatment (Song et al., 2015).

Acupuncture works on the principle of stimulating points in the body to correct imbalances in the flow of energy (qi) through channels known as meridians (Ljubinovic, 2015). Correcting imbalances in the flow of qi through the meridians in the body is based on the interaction of the five elements (wood, fire, earth, metal, and water), which have profound effects on internal organs.

One of the most common acupuncture treatments used to increase the flow of qi is known as the four gates, which involves stimulating source points on both hands between the thumb and index finger and both feet between the big toe and second toe (Errington-Evans, 2011; Ljubinovic, 2015; Eshkevari, Permaul, & Mulroney, 2003). While the four gates are commonly manipulated in acupuncture, acupuncturists will tell you that a myriad of points in the body respond to acupuncture and that any particular person will require a treatment that corresponds to that particular person's needs at a particular time.

Despite this potential variety of therapies, the four gates are part of tried-and-true treatments. One of these treatments, according to TCM, seems to be useful for tending to some mental health problems. That is because using acupuncture at the four gates counteracts symptoms that could be associated with stagnation. Physically, those symptoms could include things like constipation or menstrual cramps; psychologically, this treatment could help with people who are feeling stuck, and, therefore, those who are experiencing agitation, frustration, stress, or low mood. The four gates counteract these negative feelings because they have a powerful effect of opening up circulation throughout the body (Calabro, 2012).

SIGHT: YOGA AND MEDITATION

The Sense of Sight

If we ask ourselves what is the most striking characteristic of the visual sense, the answer might be speed. Although speed does describe the processing capacity of neurons involved in the act of seeing, these neurons act no more quickly than those used for other senses. Speed characterizes vision because the brain's visual mechanisms have to process so much while interpreting the outside environment. The other senses usually don't have to deal with so many changes at once.

If we look to our example of a primitive man again in a situation where he could be either predator or prey, we can imagine why these differences exist. In a forest, for instance, a lone human might be attentive to sounds, smells, textures, and tastes to aid him in tracking an animal. And if that lone person were to pursue that prey, the tasks of vision would suddenly become paramount in navigating the environment. Running through the trees, that individual's vision would have to constantly process the important details of an ever-changing landscape: the length and depth of depressions in the landscape; the length and strength of protruding tree branches and limbs; the moisture and arrangement of the rotting leaves on the forest floor; and the possibility of running into other animals that could be dangerous located ahead, above, and below. All this had to be taken in while dealing with a changeable environment.

The need to process this dizzying amount of information while moving through our environment might explain two interesting facts about the human sense of vision. For example, in judging the external world, the sense of depth—the three-dimensional representation of the world in our brain—is closely allied to our ability to sense motion. For objects that are stationary, our brain will often start to change the 3D image into a flatter image. One researcher speculates that this occurs because the visual "pathway [through the brain] is geared to detect changes in the environment, such as movement, and to respond quickly and briefly. Fixed on one image, its response dies out, and the impression of depth disappears."(Grady 1993) Having to take in and process multitudes of visual information simultaneously (of which depth perception is only a miniscule part) also means that our neurological system must devote a significant amount of its hardware to processing visual signals. One science writer succinctly describes how extensive this hardware is:

> The machinery that accomplishes these [visual] tasks is by far the most powerful and complex of the sensory systems. The retina, which contains 150 million light-sensitive rod and cone cells, is actually an outgrowth of the brain. In the brain itself, neurons devoted to visual processing number in the hundreds of millions and take up about 30 percent of the cortex, as compared with 8 percent for touch and just 3 percent for hearing. Each of the two optic nerves, which carry signals from the retina to the brain, consists of a million fibers; each auditory nerve carries a mere 30,000. (Grady, 1993)

One important function of vision in human development can be observed in its role in deepening the bonds and enriching the interactions between a mother and her infant child. As in breastfeeding, eye contact between a mother and her child has both physical and emotional benefits. In some studies, young mothers' feelings of anxiety about the healthy development of their children were allayed once their child began to have some sensitivity to eye contact, which happens around three to five months of age. The subliminal power of this eye contact on young mothers manifested in one study in which these women suddenly increased the amount of time they spent playing with their infants "within 2 or 3 days of [the] first recorded eye-to-eye contact, yet . . . had no idea of why this was so" (Robson, 1967). An infant's ability to recognize faces around five months of age also makes that infant's efforts to have somebody tend to his needs more efficient. In one study, researchers compared the visual interactions between babies paired with mothers and then a stranger. Babies tended to increase their vocalization or other equivalent gestures with their mothers, the people who were more likely to be responsive to their complaints (Lasky & Klein, 1979).

Sight Therapy: Yoga

Yoga helps us to leverage the sense of sight by getting the body in a relaxed state and slowing down the thinking process of the mind. In this calm state, we can use visual cues to move ourselves toward deep relaxation and, perhaps, unwind the stresses we have encountered—whether day-to-day stresses or those that span a much longer time. Much like the way a memory of an accident or particularly difficult interaction can trigger a negative emotion or feeling through the power of negative associations, so can pleasant sights and memories promote a feeling of calm and happiness. And as mentioned above, sight not only results from light entering the eye; it also is a product of the brain's very active interpretation of light data. With the brain's visual power, one can summon images almost as easily as one can passively see them. It's this power of insight that yoga can tap into.

Yoga is a 5,000-year-old practice that began in India. The word "yoga" comes from the Sanskrit root *yuj*, which means to join. In the case of yoga, the exercise attempts to join the mind, body, and spirit (Yoga.org.nz, 2015). The practice of yoga involves postures, breathing, and meditation and the benefits are intensely interwoven. As a yoga instructor and medical doctor, Timothy McCall (2007) has advocated the medicinal potential of yoga, noting that the strong and healthy postures encouraged in yoga positively affect breathing, which, in turn, can have a positive impact on one's nervous system. Yoga has many benefits that are not just physical. Some of the psychological benefits of regular yoga practice include stress reduction, increased self-awareness, less anxiety and depression, improved concentration, inner peace and calm, increased energy and vitality, and greater creativity.

Most yoga practice integrates some sort of meditation—often after the exercise session, but sometimes during the session. With eyes closed, the sensation of deep breathing helps to focus the mind. Through practice, one becomes more skilled at stepping back and observing with a nonjudging self-acceptance that helps us to recognize that we are not defined by our emotions. Internationally known meditation teacher and founder of Stress Reduction Clinic at the University of Massachusetts Medical Center, Jon Kabat-Zinn, succinctly describes yoga's potential: "When you practice yoga . . . your perspective on your body, your thoughts, and your whole sense of self can change" (1990).

For adolescents in yoga therapy sessions, yoga can be a baseline—a common denominator—from which they start to leverage visual cues. Participating together in a yoga class has the further effect of creating common experiences that adolescents can share between themselves which, it is hoped, can reinforce the lesson of insight gained through yoga.

The most visual part of yoga is the variety of poses used to exercise the body. Many of these positions are named for a physical thing that the pose resembles: Tree, Plank, Cobra, and the famous Downward-Facing Dog, just to name a few. It's an easy step to take these visually inspired poses and then use them as cues to move yoga practitioners toward a calmer state of mind. The steady effort of remaining in Downward-Facing Dog or the pleasing sense of mastery of the balance required for the Tree are some of the feelings that these yoga poses can summon. Over time, as participants in this program gain familiarity and mastery of the poses, the insights derived from them at any time during the day can become progressively easier to achieve.

APPLICATIONS

Now that we've had a bit of a whirlwind tour through the senses and the therapies that will leverage those senses, we can move to the application of this knowledge. How can we use these therapies to deal with stresses that are as alarming as they are common among our youth: stress, eating and sleeping disorders, anxiety, inability to concentrate, substance abuse, and depression? While some stress is a normal outcome of the massive amounts of physical, mental, and emotional challenges a young person must face, the scale and scope of these problems confronting our teens must shake adults out of any docile equanimity about their situation. In short, it's not okay to stand to the side and let these problems continue to buffet the lives of our children.

Luckily, there is a wealth of knowledge and experience that we can tap to help them. This first step in using that knowledge, which I've attempted in this introductory chapter, is to change our prejudices about certain medical practices, writ large: We need to stop favoring what we're familiar with (e.g., conventional medical practice) and start cultivating whatever works (ideas and insights from multiple medical systems). In the chapters that follow, I propose ways to get this process started.

CHAPTER 2

Stress

//////////////

ANNA'S DISTRACTION

I first learned about Anna in a phone call from her mother, who was concerned that her 14-year-old daughter might be suffering from depression. According to her mom, Anna exhibited a pattern of sleeping as late as possible in the morning, running out of the house without breakfast, and arriving late at school. She consistently fell asleep after midnight, and often complained about her own procrastinating as a reason for not getting her schoolwork done. She stopped spending time with friends in her limited down time and irritably complained about her siblings being immature or making too much noise.

The first time I met Anna, we spoke at length about her typical week. It was clear that she was a dedicated student who always made good grades, but she felt that she had to work harder than her peers to keep her status as a top student. She elected to take advanced placement classes because she thought it would make her a better candidate for college. When not doing homework, she spent her after-school hours at the debate club, where she was the captain, or at field hockey practice. It was clear that Anna had very little down time, or time to relax, in her busy life. Also, she admitted to having mild panic attacks before a big test, which often led to utter fatigue by the end of the day.

I felt I could help Anna create ways to cope with her frequent feelings of being overwhelmed in a way that would enable her to meet her ambitious goals. If she could use some of the integrative methods at various times during the day, I reasoned, she would hopefully learn how to bring her high-arousal state back down to baseline. We set out to develop a coping strategy that would serve her for years to come.

THE VARIETIES OF STRESSFUL CONDITIONS: NORMAL, ACUTE, AND CHRONIC STRESS

One of the most popular phrases in American English describes the condition of people who feel agitated and distracted, usually because they have too many things to do in a short amount of time: It's the feeling of being stressed out. But this term is often applied to many other kinds of stimuli that can cause feelings of distraction or distress. They can be reactions to an unwelcome surprise, like when a student just learns that her exam is coming much sooner than she had expected. Or it could be applied to a longer-term condition: to a person, for example, whose unreasonable boss causes him to fret and worry for days, weeks, or even months at a time. They all could be stressed out. As it turns out, all sorts of conditions in our lives can produce stress. In fact, feeling stress from time to time is a symptom of being alive. One early researcher in the field of stress put it this way: Complete freedom from stress is death (Seyle, 1973).

In other words, stress can be seen as a healthy adaptive response to changes in a person's life. In fact, stress is intimately connected to our development, something like growing pains. In our bodies as in our lives, there is no growth without the need to adapt—and adaptation to new or unusual circumstances can be very demanding on us. If we want to do something that requires some unusual effort—from getting up the courage to speak in public to stretching our arms as far as possible to reach for the car keys that have fallen through the floorboards of an old house—we have to ask our bodies and minds to do more than they do in a state of rest, relaxation, or equilibrium. In so doing, our bodies need extra inputs or support to function well in those times when higher demands are put on them. Let's call this normal stress.

Stress responses found in all animals can even be life saving in situations that prepare the animal to face a threat or flee to safety. In this case, chemicals and hormones are released to enhance endurance (cortisol) or alertness (epineph-rine, also known as adrenaline). We know how we feel when we are in threatening situations: The pulse quickens; breathing is faster; muscles tense; and the brain uses more oxygen and increases activity. This type of stress may even boost the immune system in the short term (National Institute of Mental Health, 2015a). These periods of greater productivity are beneficial to us and often appear before interviews, exams, or other situations where we want to succeed.

Problems with stress begin in two circumstances. The first one occurs when a specific demand at a specific time begins to put too much pressure on the body's short-term coping mechanisms. This is called acute stress. Acute stress, which is the most common form of stress, culminates from demands and pres-sures of the recent past and anticipated demands and pressures of the near future. This form of stress sometimes makes us feel thrilled and excited because it may involve challenges we choose, such as trying to get a big promotion or climbing a steep hill. But because this is short-term stress, it does not do exten-sive damage like long-term stress. Acute stress is very treatable and manage-able. According to the American Psychological Association (2015), symptoms of acute stress can include:

- *Emotional distress*—combination of the three stress emotions: anger or irrita-bility, anxiety, and depression.
- *Muscular problems* such as tension headaches, back pain, jaw pain, and mus-cular tensions that lead to pulled muscles and tendon and ligament problems.
- *Stomach, gut, and bowel problems* such as heartburn, acid stomach, flatu-lence, diarrhea, constipation, and irritable bowel syndrome.
- *Transient overarousal* that can lead to elevation in blood pressure, rapid heartbeat, sweaty palms, heart palpitations, dizziness, migraine headaches, cold hands or feet, shortness of breath, and chest pain.

Let's look in detail at a specific example of acute stress. Imagine a person marooned on a desert island who can cope with a lack of drinking water for a few days. As the amount of liquid in the body decreases, the body still needs to prioritize maintaining blood pressure and blood flow to support the important internal organs. To do this with less fluid in the body and decreased blood vol-ume, the heart rate increases and blood vessels become constricted. Eventually, this person's skin actually cools as blood is diverted from the skin for use in the internal organs. Any casual observer of this situation could notice that this person is under severe, short-term stress. While the body can succeed in keeping this poor stranded person alive for a few days, it can only do this temporarily. These kinds of extraordinary measures for survival are designed for a limited time and allow time for people under stress to search for remedies to their disequilibrium. In this case, without a remedy to a lack of drinking water—the disequilibrium, or unusual circumstance—this person will not survive.

The second kind of problematic stress is long-term or chronic stress. As emphasized in the example above, the body creates stress as a short-term remedy for some stimulus or circumstance that places unusual demands on a person. In this case, the marooned person feels stress, which is often painful and disconcerting, but eventually dies of dehydration. What would happen, however, if this person were rescued at the last minute, but his body and mind are so traumatized that they continue to act as if he is still suffering from dehydration? One could imagine that his heart rate would remain high, his skin clammy, and perhaps he would have an insatiable desire to drink water. In other words, his mechanisms for coping would be transformed from a short-term remedy to a long-term problem.

Another example of this would be the difference between reacting to a threatening situation once and reacting to that same kind of threat over days or weeks. "For the brain," one scientist writes, "the secretion of stress hormones, adrenalin and cortisol . . . in response to an acutely threatening event promotes and improves memory for the situation so that the individual can stay out of trouble in the future; yet, when the stress is repeated over many weeks, some neurons atrophy and memory is impaired, whereas other neurons grow and fear is enhanced" (McEwen, 2004). Chronic stress, then, is the condition of short-term stress being maintained for an unhealthy length of time.

Examples of chronic stress are common, such as veterans coming home from extended tours of duty suffering from post-traumatic stress disorder (PTSD). While the symptoms of PTSD vary in type and frequency depending on the individual (e.g., flashbacks, emotional withdrawal, increased arousal), the common cause is reacting as if the event that caused the trauma is still happening or may happen at any time. A battle-hardened veteran of wars abroad who becomes panicky when mistaking the sound of a car door slamming for the sound of a gunshot demonstrates how a short-term stress adaptation becomes a long-term issue for those suffering from PTSD.

There are some generalized repercussions of long-term stress. The chemicals and hormones that can be life saving in brief situations of acute stress now suppress functions that are not immediately needed. The result is lowered immunity. As a result, our digestive, excretory, and reproductive systems stop working normally. "Chronic stress appears when a person sees no way out of a miserable situation. It destroys bodies, minds, and lives" (Miller et al., 1994). Chronic stress can contribute to a wide spectrum of problems: high blood pressure, heart disease, metabolic disturbance, obesity, diabetes, insomnia, anxiety, and depression. These symptoms are often difficult to treat and sometimes require extended behavioral treatment.

STRESS AND THE ADOLESCENT POPULATION

Trying to ensure that adolescents in particular can cope with acute stress and avoid chronic stress is an important public health concern with a potentially attractive payoff. In some longitudinal studies of stress in the United States, it's been found that in general adolescents are much more susceptible to feeling stress than their parents or grandparents. The trends suggest, as we might suspect, that the perspective gained from age and experience may be crucial in helping individuals cope with stressors as they age. One researcher adds that this "interpretation is consistent with recent evidence that as people age, they focus less on negative emotions and savor positive aspects of life" (Cohen & Janicki-Deverts, 2012). This may also help to explain the importance and function of peer groups in adolescents' lives. Research has found a strong correlation between social interaction and mortality risk. A teen who feels isolated or estranged from his or her peers is left to encounter the stressors of life with limited internal coping mechanisms and outside sources of support (Holt-Lunstad, Smith, & Layton, 2010). If this is indeed the case, then reducing stress for humans at the life stage when they are most emotionally vulnerable would probably result in a significant decrease in mental health disorders faced by adult and elderly populations.

Anxiety disorders, a form of chronic stress and the most common mental illness in the United States, are widespread and costly to society (Kessler 2002). According to the most recent figures available, anxiety disorders cost the United

States more than $42 billion a year, almost one-third of the country's $148 billion total mental health bill (Hoffman 2008). Eighteen percent of the U.S. population is affected by this disorder. A national survey of adolescent mental health reported that about 8% of teens ages 13 to 18 have an anxiety disorder. Of these teens, only 18% receive mental health care (National Institute on Drug Abuse 2014; National Institute of Mental Health 2015a). Things don't seem to get much better as adolescents move on to young adulthood. Colleges across the United States report depression and anxiety as prevalent problems today. "There is no question that all of the national surveys we have at our fingertips show a distinct rise in the number of mental health problems," said Jerald Kay, professor and chair of the Department of Psychiatry at the Wright State University School of Medicine (Tartakovsky, 2008).

While the benefits of avoiding acute and chronic stress are great, the negative impact of untreated stress can be truly frightening. In some experiments conducted in the 1950s, it was found that acute stress could produce a series of serious physical problems in rats: "(1) the adrenal cortex became enlarged, (2) the thymus, spleen, lymph nodes, and all other lymphatic structures shrank, and (3) deep, bleeding ulcers appeared in the stomach and in the upper gut" (Seyle, 1973).

It is also important to note how vulnerable the brain itself is to being shaped by stress and trauma. This realization has only become widespread in the last generation. That is because as late as the 1970s, the brain was "conceived as having primarily descending influences on the body, and stressors of all varieties were thought to ignite a general and diffuse arousal reaction." But in more recent years, this paradigm of one-way communication between the brain and body has been replaced by the understanding that "the brain and body are in two-way communication via the autonomic nervous system and endocrine and immune systems." With that intense and long-term interaction, "seemingly small changes in these systems can accumulate over time." Depression, which we'll discuss in more detail later, provides an example of the negative feedback loop that can occur between the brain and body. Depression can trigger overproduction of adrenocortical hormones. In small doses, these hormones can enhance memory. In larger doses over time, these hormones can actually cause "*structural* changes [to the brain], such as atrophy of the hippocampus and hyperactivity of the amygdala" (McEwen, 2004, emphasis added).

For many adolescents, anxiety is part of the teenage years, a stage of life when many challenges take place—bodily changes, relationships with friends and parents, life goals, interests, dreams, and mental changes. Sometimes, these changes affect each other and sometimes they have nothing to do with being a teenager. In either case, the accumulation of many stressors faced during adolescence amounts to being a lot for many kids to handle.

CAUSES OF STRESS

Some of the stressors for adolescents include (Epel & Lithgow, 2014):

- *Diet:* As with the adult population, inadequate nutrient or dietary intake is a serious concern among adolescents. Poor nutritional status is stressful on the body and can contribute to a host of medical conditions. During mental and physical development, inadequate nutrition is especially damaging and can have long-term irreversible consequences.
- *Social Pressures:* Adolescents experience pressure to look or behave in certain ways or to do things because their peers are doing them. They are often exposed to risky behaviors such as underage alcohol or drug use, and may feel trapped by social expectations. Many times the peer pressures differ from what their parents recommend or demand. This results in additional tension. Moreover, mental or physical abuse may be impossible for an adolescent to talk about because of social pressures. Left untreated, the stress resulting from abuse can cause an adolescent to become isolated and have feelings of poor self-worth.
- *Illness or infection:* Any illness prompts the body to mount an immune response; the resulting healing process can be stressful and place high energy demands on the body. Chronic illnesses place an increased burden on any adolescent and can contribute to significant long-term stress.
- *Physical:* Bodily changes that alter appearance and functionality can cause stress in many ways. The unwanted changes such as pimples, vocal shifts, height, body odors, excess body hair, and the pain and inconvenience of the menstrual cycle all contribute to the awkwardness adolescents may feel with their own bodies. Sleep deprivation, a common occurrence in the adolescent

population, has been shown to elevate cortisol levels and can cause a physiological inability to remain focused, or even look healthy.

- *Psychological:* The ideals of adolescents begin to change and no longer align with the parental ideals they were raised with and, as a result, parents become concerned. Choice of religion or political ideas may change with an adolescent as new discoveries are made. Sexual orientation is another discovery that may not gain parental approval, which can cause the adolescent to feel unloved and misunderstood.

- *Other stressors:* Difficulty in school, trouble meeting and making new friends, keeping up with fashion and trends, all can further contribute to stress and anxiety. Not having the funds to join in interests with others or the inability to join sports or other activities because an after-school job is necessary can also be contributing factors.

PHYSIOLOGY OF THE STRESS RESPONSE

As discussed above, stress can occur in many forms. No matter the type, it elicits the body's stress response, which initiates a cascade of stress hormones, cytokines, and inflammatory mediators. Physiologically, the fight-or-flight response is triggered during a perceived threat. It allows our system to respond, avert danger, and return to baseline. Certain chronic situations can expose the body to extended periods of excessive stress and contribute to long-term negative health effects. When a person is experiencing chronic stress, the body attempts to develop coping mechanisms. The brain, the organ that responds to stress, determines what the threat is and what type of physiological responses could be damaging. During this process, the brain communicates with cardiovascular, immune, and other systems in the body via neural and endocrine mechanisms (McEwen, 2004).

When a person confronts perceived danger, the eyes or ears send the information to the amygdala (area of brain contributing to emotional processing). The amygdala interprets the images and sounds and instantly sends a distress signal to the hypothalamus (the area of the brain that functions like a command center), communicating with the rest of the body through the nervous system so the person has the energy to fight or flee.

In essence, the amygdala sends a distress signal; the hypothalamus activates the sympathetic nervous system by sending signals through the autonomic nerves to the adrenal glands. These glands respond by pumping the hormone epinephrine into the bloodstream. As epinephrine circulates through the body, it brings on a number of physiological changes that happen very quickly:

- The heart beats faster than normal, pushing blood to the muscles, heart, and other vital organs.
- Pulse rate and blood pressure go up.
- The person undergoing these changes begins to breathe more rapidly, causing extra oxygen to be sent to the brain, increasing alertness.
- Sight, hearing, and other senses become sharper.
- Epinephrine triggers release of blood sugar (glucose) and fats from storage sites in the body and supply energy to all parts of the body.

The hypothalamus releases corticotrophin-releasing hormone, which travels to the pituitary gland, triggering the release of adrenocorticotrophic hormone. This hormone then travels to the adrenal glands, prompting them to release cortisol. When the threat passes, cortisol levels fall and the parasympathetic nervous system then dampens the stress response (Dusek et al., 2008; Holt-Lunstad et al., 2010).

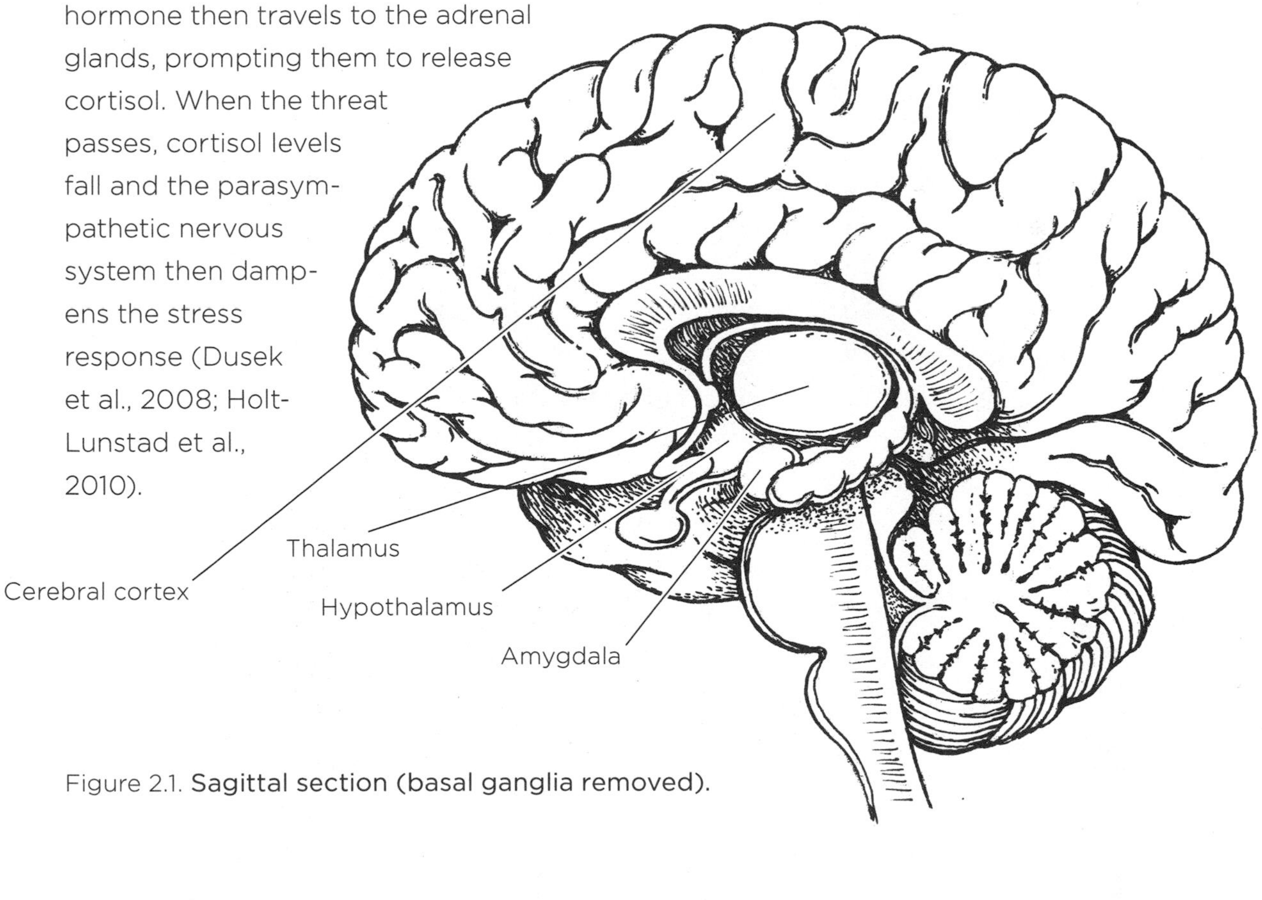

Cerebral cortex

Thalamus

Hypothalamus

Amygdala

Figure 2.1. **Sagittal section (basal ganglia removed).**

SIGNS AND SYMPTOMS OF STRESS

Preteens and adolescents often find stressful situations associated with making and keeping friendships, achieving in school, and trying to live up to perceived expectations from parents, teachers, or coaches. During times of chronic stress, emotional symptoms can appear as acting out, agitation, depression, nervousness, anxiousness, fearfulness, or feelings of being under constant pressure. The person may suffer from emotional breakdowns. Symptoms of stress and anxiety can often be experienced as an ominous feeling or sense of impending doom, negative thoughts, physical illness, or behavioral actions such as restlessness or uncharacteristic aggression.

Adults are not always aware when their children or teens are experiencing overwhelming feelings of stress. Recognizing the signs of stress in a child or teen is important for parents if they are to offer guidance and support to their children. A few signs of stress may include:

1. *Negative changes in behavior.* These are almost always an indication that something is wrong. A parent can suspect stress if a child or teen is acting irritable or moody, withdrawing from activities that used to give him or her pleasure, expressing worries, complaining more than usual about school, crying, displaying surprising fearful reactions, clinging to a parent or teacher, sleeping too much or too little, or eating too much or too little. Additionally, stress may be the culprit when teens abandon longtime friendships for a new set of peers, or express hostility toward family members (American Psychological Association, 2015).

2. *Physical symptoms.* Physical signs of significant stress usually include stomachaches and headaches, especially if a physician previously gave the child a clean bill of health.

3. *Poor interaction with others.* While a child or teen may seem just fine at home, this may not be the case in other settings. It is important for parents to network with other parents to understand how the child or teen is doing in the outside world. Communication with other parents, teachers, and coaches of extracurricular activities may help parents to understand what their children are thinking or feeling. It may also bring awareness to any sources of concern.

4. *Troubling Words.* These can include "worried," "confused," "annoyed," and "angry." If you are hearing these words from your child or teen, be concerned and try to understand what may be happening to cause your child or teen to use these words.

BAD COPING MECHANISMS FOR STRESS

Our emotions also get involved with stress relief. Unfortunately, not all coping mechanisms are healthy. In some cases, negative coping responses for short-term emotional stress relief can bring on other complications that can make the patient's overall health worse. These coping strategies—such as alcohol, drugs, caffeine, or overeating—are as unhelpful as they are popular. Because of their connection to our emotions, these bad habits can create considerable obstacles to effective therapies and, therefore, deserve some consideration.

Food, for instance, is often used as way to comfort or distract people who are experiencing stressful situations. This phenomenon is so large that a popular term is attached to it that most of us have heard: emotional eating. Some factors that contribute to bad eating habits include low self-esteem and low levels of social support, as well as stress. One unhealthy coping mechanism, avoidant coping, is closely associated with bad eating behaviors. And many unhealthy cycles can commence with eating due to stress: "high fatty food consumption, decreased fruit and vegetable intake, and decreased breakfast consumption among adolescents" (Martyn-Nemeth, Penckofer, Gulanick, Velsor-Friedrich, & Bryant, 2009).

As adolescents move to college age, one coping mechanism they often turn to is drinking alcohol. Younger adolescents can turn to drinking as well, but alcohol is much easier to access as adolescents move away from living with their parents. It also becomes more central to their social lives. Like bad eating habits, drinking can be associated with avoidance coping, at least in general. One researcher has found that while there may not be a one-to-one correlation with avoidance coping and drinking, the use of avoidance coping as a strategy for dealing with stress could "[exacerbate] ongoing problems over time, leading to higher levels of negative mood, which in turn are associated with increased drinking" (Park, Armell, & Tennen, 2004).

As mentioned previously, there are different kinds of stress; and, even more importantly, there are many kinds of symptoms of stress that, left untreated, can lead to permanent and debilitating conditions. In the case of drinking or eating as a coping mechanism for stress, these bad strategies are not only ineffective, but they also lead to deepening degrees of other problems in a process that might be described as a vicious cycle. The alternative therapies described in this book may be able to mitigate the problems brought on by bad habits; moreover, these therapies may also get adolescents on the path of creating their own virtuous cycles of health and happiness. The goal of this chapter is to describe ways to diminish stress in general and, in some cases, get adolescents on a healthier path to overall progress and well-being in their mental health.

TREATMENT PROTOCOLS AND SUPPORTIVE THERAPIES

It is important for people from every age group to find that balance between body, mind, emotions, and behavior. This is true whether or not stress is involved. In addition to pharmaceutical therapy for stress, social and behavioral interventions such as regular physical activity and social support can help to reduce the chronic stress burden and benefit brain and body health and resilience (McEwen, 2004).

There are many techniques that people can learn to help them counter the stress response such as relaxation, physical activity, and social support. These techniques are quite successful as a counter to stress when used in combination (Dusek et al., 2008; Holt-Lunstad et al., 2010; McEwen, 2002).

- *Relaxation response.* Deep abdominal breathing, focus on a soothing word such as "peace" or "calm," visualization of tranquil scenes, repetitive prayers, yoga, and tai chi are just a few of the approaches that can be used to prompt the relaxation response. While these approaches are not a cure-all for most people with severe stress, they are beneficial.
- *Physical activity.* Exercise is often recommended to people who complain of stress. This activity is also beneficial to children and teens. Physical exercise such as brisk walking that increases the heart rate helps to relieve muscle tension caused by stress. Movement therapies including yoga, tai chi, and qigong combine fluid movements with deep breathing and mental focus

to create calm. For children and teens, any physical activity such as after-school sports can provide exercise, as well as social support.

- *Social support.* Peer relationships, friendships, coworker communications, spouses, and daily companions provide necessary daily enhancements. People who have close relationships with family and friends garner emotional support that definitely helps them during times of stress.

- *Other therapies* such as acupuncture, TCM, Ayurvedic medicine (use of herbal diets and other compounds), massage therapy, relaxation, and music or sound therapy have shown success in stress management (Hanley, Stirling, & Brown, 2003; Dixit, Agrawal, & Dubey, 1993; Richardson & Rothstein, 2008).

- *Nutrition.* Research has shown that the human body depletes stores of nutrients such as protein and vitamins B, C, and A when under stress. According to Holistic Online.com, prolonged stress or a risk of hypertension can often be countered by consuming foods high in potassium (orange juice, squash, potatoes, apricots, limes, bananas, avocados, tomatoes, peaches). Other foods that can be beneficial during times of high stress include yogurt, cheese, tofu, and chickpeas.

HELPING ANNA

Anna and I worked together, using a toolbox approach to adaptive interventions. We created a schedule for the following: music therapy, abdominal breathing, acupressure, yoga, and aromatherapy.

We sketched out a typical day for her, adding time for the various therapies. Mornings were clearly very difficult for Anna. She told me that when she woke up the first thing she thought about was all the homework she didn't finish the night before, and started spinning her wheels trying to think of ways to make up the lost time. So I asked her to start a routine of putting on music that she found uplifting but not too energetic. (She chose artists such as Adele, Sam Smith, etc.) Anna agreed that the first thing she would usually do when she woke up was to think about her homework. But her second action would be to put on the selected music. She was allowed to lie in bed listening for 10 minutes, and she could keep the music on while getting dressed.

To address moments of anxiety throughout the day, Anna learned how to take a 5-minute time-out to do deep abdominal breathing. To find privacy for this activity, she identified two locations at the school where she could go: the bathroom and the cafeteria when not in use. If a location was not available, she would use acupressure wherever she was at a given time. For example, she could use her forefinger to press an acupoint on the wrist (PC6, described in protocol section for this chapter) thought to be useful in bringing the mind back to the present, inducing a sense of calm, and directing the mind away from troubling thoughts.

Her bedtime routine focused on calming her nervous system and slowing down her body and mind. Just before getting into bed, Anna would do a series of forward bends on her bedroom floor. Poses such as Standing Forward Pose and Downward-Facing Dog were used to promote sleepiness. Then, after climbing into bed and turning out the light, Anna would place on her pillow near her nose a sachet bag steeped in lavender, a flower known for its calming fragrance.

Anna agreed to try these interventions for one week, and then we would meet again to check in. After the first week of self-therapy, Anna reported that she was not improving overall, but did feel a little more in control now that she had something to focus on, as if the therapies were a welcome distraction in the course of a typical day. I considered that a sign of early progress, and we agreed that she would continue her routines and we would meet again in two weeks.

At the one-month mark, Anna was feeling a slight reduction in generalized anxiety. By the end of her sessions at the clinic, Anna was reporting having deeper sleep—even more dreams—and also waking up half an hour earlier in the morning. Her ability to get through the school day was improving, she said, but she also wanted to explore more interventions in the future, such as acupuncture, and begin a regular exercise routine.

CHAPTER 2 STRESS SENSORY TREATMENT PROTOCOL*

Touch: Acupressure Points**—GV20, Yintang, and PC6

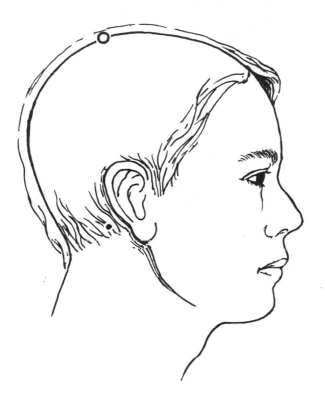

GV20

In TCM the governing vessel (GV) or channel is thought to supply the brain and spinal regions. This point is located approximately 5 cun*** back along the scalp from the hairline.

*Please refer to the Treatment Protocol Information and Resource Guide of this book (page 197) for additional detailed information on how to self-administer all sensory treatments and for added resources to locate these integrative therapies online and in local communities.

**For all acupressure points: Once you locate the point, stimulate it by pressing down with your index or middle finger and provide moderate pressure. Rotate your finger in a circular motion while pressing over the point. Continue to stimulate or massage the area for 2–3 minutes. Can be repeated as needed.

***A cun is a unit of measurement in TCM that refers to the width of the patient's thumb.

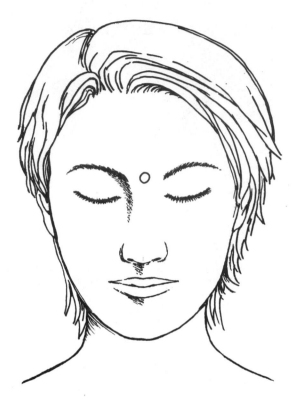

Yintang

The yintang point is located in the midline between the eyebrows. It is found on what is called an extraordinary (EX) meridian or channel in TCM. These EX meridians include acupoints (locations for acupressure or acupuncture) that are not on the 14 main channels. This point has been used in CAM treatment to reduce tension, ease headache, and provide relief from sinus congestion.

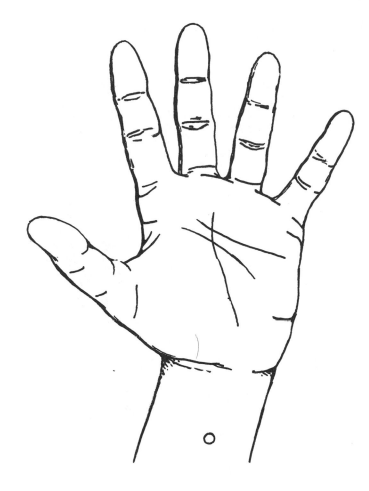

PC6

This point is located on the pericardium (PC) channel. It can be found approximately 2 cun proximal to the crease of the wrist. Acupoints on the limbs (arms and legs) are bilateral. So while they may be shown on one side of the body, they have bilateral application.

Smell: Herbs, Flowers, Plants, and Essential Oils*—Lavender and Rose

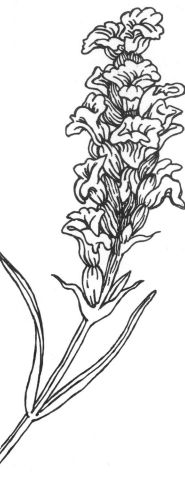

Lavender (*Lavandula officinalis*)

Lavender is an herb native to France and the western Mediterranean. It was often used in ancient Roman baths as a way to cleanse body and soul—thus its name coming from the Latin word *lavare*, which means "to wash." This perennial shrub is now cultivated worldwide for both medicinal and perfume use. It became popular in the Middle Ages for medicinal applications of stress, tension, and ailments of the brain. Small studies suggest that it has indeed worked for problems like anxiety and insomnia.

*Essential Oils (EO) have several methods of use. Please refer to the Treatment Protocol Information and Resource Guide of this book (page 197) for additional detailed information on aromatherapy.

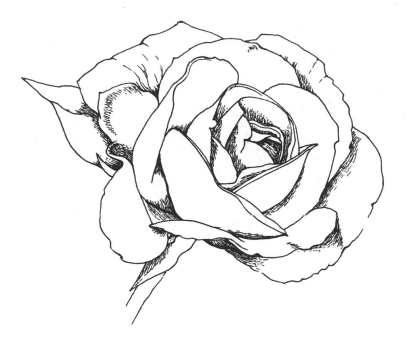

Rose (*Rosa damascena***)**

Rose has a long history and appears in ancient Ayurvedic texts. There is preliminary evidence from animal models and small-scale human studies that rose oil has reduced stress and tension. While larger human studies are needed, it appears rose oil can have a supportive role and work as an adjuvant with other stress-relieving therapies.

Taste: Herbal Tisanes*—Chamomile, Lemon Balm

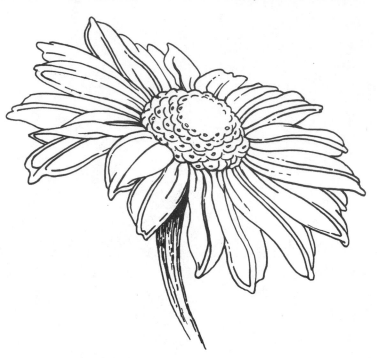

Chamomile (*Anthemis nobilis* and *Matricaria chamomilla*)

Chamomile has been used as a calming agent for centuries and is very safe. Even the ancient Egyptians considered it a prized herb for a host of medical conditions. There are two types: Roman (*Anthemis nobilis*) and German (*Matricaria chamomilla*); both have calming properties. The flower heads of the plant are used for the herbal tisane.

Chamomile has a long history of use as an anti-inflammatory, antispasmodic, and anxiolytic. It has also been used for digestive disorders and nervous tension. Conditions such as muscle spasms, stomachaches, and menstrual cramps can be alleviated, too.

It's effective and mild at the same time, which is why it can be so useful. For instance, in a baby with colic, chamomile can at once deal with the digestive problem while also soothing the baby to prepare it for sleep.

*Tea and herbal tisanes are easy to prepare and find at local stores and markets. For detailed information on preparation and sourcing please refer to the Treatment Protocol Information and Resource Guide on page 197.

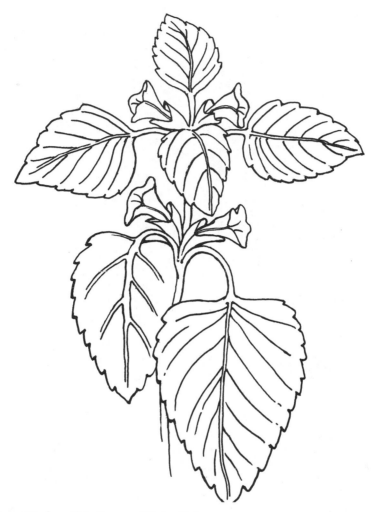

Lemon Balm (*Melissa officinalis***)**

This herb is native to southern Europe, western Asia, and northern Africa. Lemon balm's botanical name, *Melissa*, originates from the Greek word for "bee." This is in reference to the strong attraction these insects have for the plant.

In medieval times the herb was valued to such a degree, both for its beauty and healing properties, that Emperor Charlemagne ordered the plant be grown in all monastery gardens. Monks began using the herb for many different health purposes, not only as a tisane but also a protective salve.

Preliminary research shows lemon balm can help reduce anxiety and stress in children and adults (Cases, 2010; Pardo-Aldave et al., 2009).

Sight: Yoga Postures—Lotus Pose, Child's Pose, and Seated Forward Bend

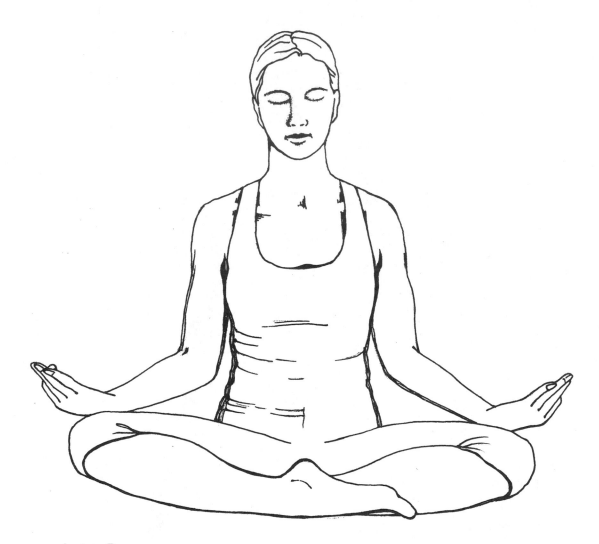

Lotus Pose

This pose opens the hips and creates a sense of balance. It is one of the most historic poses in ancient yoga practice. Start by sitting with both legs straight in front of you. Next, bend your right knee and bring the heel of the foot into the inner thigh of the left. Then lift the left foot and bend the left knee gently toward the right inner thigh. This is a more relaxed version of the pose. There are more difficult variations, but this is a good place to start.

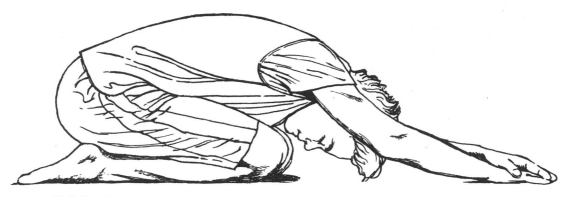

Child's Pose

This position stretches your lower back and arms as well as relaxing the entire body. It increases circulation to the head. If you have knee problems, use caution when lowering the body. Slide your buttocks toward your heels and stretch your body downward. Once in a fully stretched position, rest your arms fully in front of you and rest your stomach on your knees. Allow your body to ease into this stretch by keeping the arms and neck relaxed.

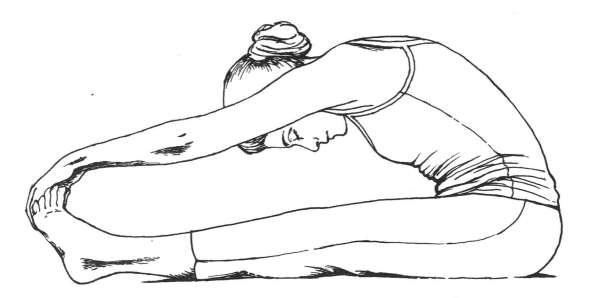

Seated Forward Bend

This is a basic pose that can be done in more challenging ways depending on your skill level and familiarity with yoga. Start in a seated position on the floor. Sit up straight with your legs stretched out in front of you. Inhale as you stretch your arms up over your head. Exhale as you bend forward and stretch out toward your feet with your hands. If you can touch your feet, take hold of your big toes with your index fingers. A more relaxed version is to grasp the toes with your hands with feet pointing upward. This pose benefits the hamstrings and stretches and lengthens the spine.

Sound: Relaxing Music, Including Slow-Tempo, Soothing Nature, and Earth Sounds

For relaxation, the most beneficial sounds include those with slow melodies and depth and songs that use lower frequencies and slow transitions. Nature sounds such as rain or water have consistent frequencies, or white noise, which has a calming effect on the nervous system. Smooth sounds with gentle transitions are relaxing and ease tension.

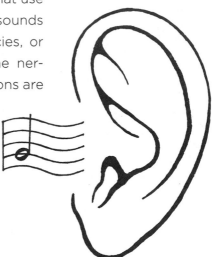

CHAPTER 3

Fatigue

////////////////

MEET CARLOS

There are a lot of different reasons for adolescents to feel fatigue, and a wide variety of kids who come to my clinics feel like they just don't have enough energy. One typical profile for a student complaining of fatigue is the high achiever. These are kids who try to excel on many levels. I got to know one high school student just like this: Carlos. He was a sweet kid, always presenting himself well in public, well dressed and well spoken. And he would surprise people with wry comments now and then that could make everybody laugh.

Although he was generally upbeat, he was also under a lot of pressure. He was pushing himself mentally and physically. Academically, he was striving to do his best and had enrolled in a lot of advanced placement, or college-level, classes. He also was involved in a lot of extracurricular activities: writing and taking photos for the school yearbook as well as participating in the swim team. It was his senior year, so he was also applying to colleges. Simultaneously, his family was dealing with financial difficulties. Being the good son that he was, he was also working at a job to contribute to the family income.

Adolescents like Carlos are pushing themselves to the limit on so many different levels. They're staying up late to finish assignments while they're applying to college, burning the candle at both ends to complete applications. Or they're overextended in general. In addition to sports and school, they have lots of social commitments. What often happens is that they put a premium on doing things quickly and don't pay attention to the body's basic needs. They're not getting a lot of sleep and they're not eating or hydrating very well, so their nutritional status is not where it should be. There's a whole host of reasons contributing to the body just feeling depleted, so it's no surprise that they feel tired. What compounds this is that they're often mentally and physically spent, and the two conditions can work together to further deepen their fatigue.

If you keep accommodating this kind of unreasonable schedule, more bad things can happen. For Carlos it was his diet, which was terrible. Everything he ate was fast food, really poor-quality stuff. In addition to very poor sleep, he wasn't getting the nutrition he needed. Adding the stress of his personal responsibilities, it was a perfect storm that made him mentally and physically depleted.

The body needs to replenish at some point, but these high achievers typically don't allow that to happen. When I first met Carlos, he dragged himself into my office and sat down with a heavy thud. He tried to put a smile on his lackluster presence, but it was clear that he was running out of resources to deal with the demanding schedule he set for himself. Fortunately, the advice and direction he got from the clinic helped him to get back into balance.

WHAT IS FATIGUE?

The consensus among scientists who study fatigue is that there is no consensus about fatigue. What it is exactly, its origins, and its impacts have not all been precisely delineated. One emerging line of argument is that fatigue is a combination of physical and emotional states that arise when the costs we incur to achieve a goal begin to exceed the expected rewards. The purpose of fatigue in this view, then, can be seen as being the body's attempt to conserve energy (Ekkekakis, Hargreaves, & Parfitt, 2013; Boksem & Tops, 2008).

While examining the potential causes of fatigue is important in the effort to diagnose fatigue and prescribe remedies for it (which we will explore in the following pages), I use a simple working definition that will enable us to get started with the task at hand: helping adolescents who feel like they don't have the resources to deal with their daily tasks and responsibilities. For adolescents complaining of these symptoms, fatigue can be understood as a feeling of tiredness or a lack of energy that can be improved by sleep and/or rest. Once a doctor or clinician comes to the conclusion that an adolescent is dealing with this simple version of fatigue, attending to the symptoms can be relatively straightforward (although execution of the prescription may sometimes be challenging). To keep a clear idea about what fatigue is, one must also maintain a distinction between fatigue and sleepiness. According to one researcher, sleepiness is "'an increased tendency to fall asleep' and is generally considered the opposite of alertness" (Findlay, 2008). So while a sleepy person and a fatigued person may complain of feeling tired, the actions that are associated with that tired feeling (falling asleep versus feeling depleted) are different.

And before coming to the conclusion that a patient is suffering from fatigue, a clinician faces a much more important task: examining other conditions that could have fatigue as a symptom. For instance, it's important to distinguish between fatigue, as we've defined it, and chronic fatigue or chronic fatigue syndrome. Chronic fatigue is defined as "self-reported persistent or relapsing fatigue lasting 6 or more consecutive months" (Fukada et al., 1994). Because this is a medical condition that encompasses a more extensive and pervasive constellation of symptoms, it merits an assessment by a physician. In this situation, the fatigue is severe and not relieved by bed rest. It may involve several body systems and include muscle aches and weakness, difficulty concentrating, and memory impairment. Moreover, although fatigue and chronic fatigue have many similarities, dealing with the two conditions requires very different protocols. Unlike fatigue, chronic fatigue does not improve with or respond to better patterns of rest and sleep. Luckily, this is not a very common malady faced by adolescents.

While fatigue in many cases may not be a sign of chronic fatigue syndrome, it can sometimes be a sign of some other serious mental or physical condition, some of which include pulmonary diseases, diabetes, cardiac problems, kidney failure, lupus, and multiple sclerosis, among other causes. When enough sleep, good nutrition, or a low-stress environment does not relieve fatigue, fatigue could also be a sign of clinical depression (Ekkekakis et al., 2013).

Fatigue can also be divided into two distinct camps: mental and physical fatigue. While the two are different, they can often exist simultaneously in the same person. Imagine somebody struggling through the middle of a challenging outdoor ropes or obstacle course. While expending a lot of physical energy moving through the course, one also has to decide the best path through it, thinking before leaping, if you will. Nevertheless, the two actions are distinct. For mental fatigue, some interpretations of the phenomenon see it as a result of a person doing some sort of mental work that will not result in a satisfactory reward. Contrary to what may seem like common sense, mental fatigue does not correlate with the amount of mental effort spent (perhaps best measured in continuous thinking and/or concentration). If the rewards seem great, people can concentrate on a mental task for an extended time without feeling fatigue.

Similarly, in the case of physical fatigue, there is no absolute correlation between the perceived amount of exertion and tiredness of the muscles or circulatory system. Instead, there is a steep decline in the feeling of pleasure experienced by a person during physical exertion. While the degree of the feeling of pleasure is indeed associated with physical changes occurring during exercise, the key trigger for feeling fatigue seems to be a decrease in the amount of pleasure associated with that exercise. This phenomenon, writes one researcher, "is the main vehicle by which critical departures from homeostatic balance enter into consciousness" (Ekkekakis et al., 2013).

The close associations between mental states like pleasure and pain as well as effort and reward with feelings of fatigue reinforces the understanding of the importance of the brain in shaping human beings' perceptions of themselves. The ways these feelings enter our consciousness are indeed subtle and multi-layered. When a feeling like fatigue becomes too pervasive in our day-to-day lives, holistic approaches to improving mental health tend to the subtlety of the human interior life with gentle and gently progressive therapies, thus promising to correct the main problem (in this case, fatigue) without creating other problems as a side effect of therapy.

PHYSIOLOGY OF FATIGUE

While mental fatigue may, in the end, result from a subjective cost-benefit analysis, the sources of physical fatigue are a little easier to pin down—although many unresolved questions about fatigue remain.

Physical fatigue resulting from exertion might be placed in three broad categories: episodic fatigue, chronic fatigue, and disease- or malady-related illness. In the first category, we would find things related to energy output, like intense exercise or perhaps a high-stress situation that results in exhaustion. Fatigue could also be related to a disequilibrium in energy input, such as dehydration or a temporary lack of nutrition. The second category of fatigue relates to more long-term problems. The most well-known is chronic fatigue syndrome, mentioned above. Finally, fatigue can be a clear symptom of other chronic conditions, as well as health problems that are often shorter term, such as cancer and anemia.

The physiological and metabolic causes of fatigue are varied; often, more than one of these causes can affect a particular patient. As one researcher has summarized, "Fatigue from exertion may be related to deconditioning (decreased maximal cardiac output and/or reduced muscle perfusion or oxidative capacity), reduced muscle mass or muscle quality, anemia, poor oxygen extraction [from the blood to the body], [or] poor nutrition or malnutrition" (Evans & Lambert, 2007). Ongoing research suggests that changes in rehabilitative regimes related to fatigue as a symptom of illness may need to be made. It may be that those rehabilitating from cancer, for example, might decrease their feeling of fatigue by beginning guided exercise programs during cancer treatment. As William Evans points out, only recently those who had suffered from heart attacks were advised to undergo extensive bed rest. Now, more vigorous means to enable cardiac rehabilitation is the standard of care (Evans & Lambert, 2007).

SIGNS AND SYMPTOMS OF FATIGUE

Fatigue signs and symptoms may be physical, mental, or emotional in nature (Medical News Today, 2015):

- Bloating, abdominal pain, constipation, diarrhea, nausea, possible problems similar to irritable bowel syndrome
- Aching or sore muscles
- Painful lymph nodes
- Apathy, lack of motivation
- Chronic tiredness
- Difficulty concentrating
- Dizziness
- Hallucinations

- Impaired hand-to-eye coordination
- Headache
- Impaired judgment
- Indecisiveness
- Irritability
- Loss of appetite
- Moodiness
- Poor immune system function
- Sleepiness, drowsiness
- Slower than normal reflexes

BAD COPING MECHANISMS FOR FATIGUE

Poor coping mechanisms to deal with fatigue are well known. Many people try to use some sort of stimulant to force themselves through fatigue to get their day's work done, including cigarettes, drugs, energy drinks, and caffeine. Conversely, some people try to suppress or ignore fatigue by pretending it doesn't exist (also known as avoidance coping). Avoidance may also include habits like drinking alcohol, which does help people fall asleep but robs them of an important portion of their REM cycle, thus making their sleep much less restorative. For those trying to suppress fatigue, their bottled-up feelings and emotions often come out unexpectedly through emotional outbursts, which often puzzle and alarm people they live and work with. These outbursts ratchet up any existing tensions with others, thus adding to conditions that may promote bad sleeping habits.

Left unchecked, it is possible these bad coping mechanisms can turn the minor problem of fatigue into the more serious condition of chronic fatigue syndrome. One study of nurses working the late shift suggested that suppressive coping mechanisms for fatigue "significantly predicted chronic fatigue" (Samaha, Lal, Samaha, & Wyndham, 2007).

FATIGUE AND ADOLESCENTS

About 30% of adolescents report some feeling of fatigue after expending energy for normal activity (Fisher, 2003). In comparison, about 20% of adults up to age

65 complain of feeling fatigue (Blackwell & Clarke, 2013). While that represents a large percentage of the adolescent population, it does not mean that adolescents need a significantly different amount of sleep than other age groups. Contrary to what might be popularly believed, adolescents do not need much more sleep than younger kids do. What is different, though, is the rhythms by which they sleep and the problems caused by those changed rhythms. Studies have shown that the circadian rhythms of kids hitting puberty start to shift 2 hours later (meaning a later ideal bedtime and waking time than before). So elementary school kids who might be bright and happy when the 8:00 A.M. bell rings turn into much more tired, grumpy, and distracted teenagers heading to school at the same time. These changes are exacerbated by other influences that can tend to keep adolescents up later: more school activities, more homework, more screen time (both TV and video games), and clandestine late-night communication with friends via some form of social media. Unfortunately, sleeping more on the weekend can't make up for lost opportunities for sleep during the school week. In fact, the difference between weekend and school week sleeping, some researchers have speculated, may give kids feelings similar to jet lag at the beginning of the week (Fisher, 2003).

One interesting research study (not yet conclusive) suggests that there may be significant differences in the rates of fatigue among adolescent boys and girls. This study, performed in the Netherlands, showed that girls consistently registered more instances of feeling fatigue than did boys (ter Wolbeek, van Doornen, Kavelaars, & Heijnen, 2006). For example, while 16.4% of girls reported feeling severe fatigue for more than a month, only 4.0% of boys reported feeling the same kind of fatigue. The reasons behind this have not been found conclusively, but one study points to the possibility that "a higher sensitivity in stimulus processing develops during adolescence" for girls (Davis, Matthews, & Twamley, 1990). In addition to possibly perceiving "events as more stressful," girls may also be exposed to more stressful situations. This increased stress among girls could be related to different rates of fatigue in boys and girls.

TREATMENT PROTOCOLS AND SUPPORTIVE THERAPIES

The first step in dealing with fatigue or fatigue symptoms is to check for any other underlying medical condition. If not, the next thing to do is to have patients jot down their daily routine. They should answer questions such as, What time do you get up? What time do you go to bed? What occurs during your day? This will give you a list of their daily activities and when they occur. This helps us get an idea of exactly what they are cramming into their day, and how much sleep and downtime they are giving themselves.

Ultimately, we need to determine the patient's sleep/wake cycle (circadian rhythm) because that's one of the most basic bodily functions—the downtime to restore. If you see early on that a healthy sleep cycle is missing from an adolescent's life, you know that many other things are off-kilter as well. Why? Because we know from studies that even two to three nights of sleep deprivation shoots up cortisol levels. The result is a state of increased stress. Add that to that lack of restorative sleep, and then feeling worn out and exhausted is the next step. If we can stop these habits before they get too ingrained, long-term damage can be easily avoided. But more serious issues, especially chronic fatigue syndrome, could result from bad sleeping habits that are left unchecked.

Tending to fatigue is so dependent on the source and what's going on in a person's life. If it is a simple version of fatigue due to mental or physical overexertion, usually adolescents will start to feel effects of treatment within a week—if they're really sticking with the program. That means starting to give themselves adequate sleep, engaging in some downtime during the day, and getting less mental or physical stimulation right before sleep.

Once the underlying cause of fatigue is found, treatment can begin:

- *Anemia or low iron without anemia:* iron supplements
- *Sleep apnea:* specific medications and medical devices
- *Blood sugar:* medications to regulate blood sugar levels
- *Underactive thyroid:* targeted pharmacological therapy
- *Obesity:* diet and exercise regimen
- *Depression or grief:* counseling, psychotherapy, pharmacologic agents
- *Persistent pain:* physical therapy, acupuncture, herbal remedies, electrical stimulation devices, trigger point injections, pharmacologic agents
- *Fibromyalgia:* physical therapy, relaxation techniques, psychological and behavioral therapy, herbal remedies, pharmacologic agents

Treatments to help reduce fatigue might include the following:

- Getting enough sleep each night
- Eating a healthy, well-balanced diet and drinking plenty of water throughout the day
- Exercising regularly
- Learning better ways to relax such as yoga or meditation
- Maintaining a reasonable work and personal schedule
- Reducing life stressors
- Avoiding alcohol, nicotine, and drug use

HELPING CARLOS

When I first met Carlos, he was at the end of his rope, so to speak, and was finally ready to change his habits. The first thing we taught him is that good sleep is crucial to good health. It's so restorative. A whole host of hormones are released during sleep. Further, important brain functions that include memory consolidation and learning as well as immune responses that help the body fight infection occur, specifically during sleep, so people need to let themselves rest. Unless you give sleep its due, you can't perform your daily tasks the way you'd like to.

Of course, we have a series of sensory treatments that can be helpful for kids like Carlos. But before we get to any of them, we have to do something even more crucial. We need our patient to commit to changing his sleep habits. People who like to see themselves as energetic and maybe even indestructible have a hard time saying, "Enough! I really need to slow down." Nevertheless, I demanded that if Carlos was going to embark on this effort to lessen his fatigue, he had to put into place a good program for sleep hygiene. As busy as he was, I was asking him to carve out another piece of his day to get better sleep. But if there's any point in your life when you're going to give yourself time to replenish, this has got to be it. So, in this student's case, after he made this active commitment, the next step was just putting him on a healthier plan.

So how do you get a teenager to fall asleep earlier? Every parent knows you can mandate a certain bedtime or lights-out time, but you can't force a teenager to fall asleep early. It's like forcing a child to eat—there's only so much pleading and coercing you can do. In the end, the child has all the control. Thankfully, there are ways to appeal to a teenager's sense of self and self-image when teaching the benefits of sleep. I explain to my clients that during sleep, various hormones and antioxidants are released that make the skin more radiant. This is true, and it can be anecdotally verified by looking at yourself in a mirror after you've had 4 hours of sleep versus 9. I also point out that good sleep promotes the consolidation of muscle memory. So if you are learning a new football play, for example, the brain will more quickly integrate what's learned during the day if it gets a solid amount of sleep at night. In short, good sleep promotes better learning. This line of reasoning may at first sound devious or opportunistic, but it is factually accurate and resonates with teenagers' developmentally appropriate values. After I get the patient's agreement and commitment to change sleeping habits, the next step is to provide the tools to help wind down in the evening and set the stage for relaxation and sleep.

For Carlos, the plan was pretty easy to follow. He had to commit to a relatively early time to go to bed so he could get a good amount of sleep, which means 8–10 hours for an adolescent. Eating well was important too. We had to make sure that he had breakfast. He was not a breakfast eater, so he sometimes wouldn't eat anything until one in the afternoon. This habit would exhaust him in the morning and then encourage him to eat just any convenient (and often unhealthy) thing that was easily available.

In addition to changing his sleep and eating habits, we also added a brief pause in his day through a relaxation technique. It was pretty simple: He would just find 10 minutes a day at least to slow down. And slowing down could be done in a variety of ways: placing himself in a yoga position, lying down to take a catnap, or manipulating an acupressure point. Anything that helps the patient center himself and cut out the noise of his daily schedule is productive.

Finally, I asked Carlos to keep a very minimal sleep diary. He recorded sleep and wake times, and indicated whether it felt restorative or not. It's important to keep it simple for busy teenagers, because asking for too much documentation will turn them away.

To Carlos's surprise, he started to feel better within a week. He could focus better, had more energy to engage in all of his activities, and just generally felt better throughout the day. So Carlos's issues weren't particularly difficult to fix. Just two things were needed: a strong personal commitment and also a multifaceted approach. In Carlos's case, you couldn't just deal with sleep and ignore diet or vice versa. He had to be helped in a multimodal way.

CHAPTER 3 FATIGUE SENSORY TREATMENT PROTOCOL*

Touch: Acupressure Points** ST36, SP6, LV3

ST36 (Stomach Channel)
With a slightly flexed knee, this point is found on the shin approx 3 cun (three thumb widths) below the patella and just outside (lateral to) the prominent tibia bone.

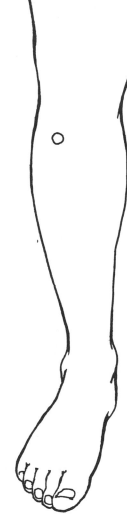

*Please refer to the Treatment Protocol Information and Resource Guide of this book (page 197) for additional detailed information on how to self-administer all sensory treatments and for added resources to locate these integrative therapies online and in local communities.

**For all acupressure points: Once you locate the point, stimulate it by pressing down with your index or middle finger and provide moderate pressure. Rotate your finger in a circular motion while pressing over the point. Continue to stimulate or massage the area for 2–3 minutes. Can be repeated as needed.

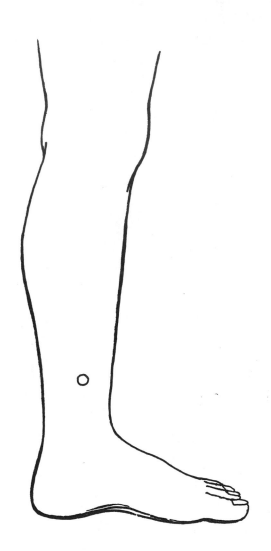

SP6 (Spleen Channel)

Located on the inside of the lower leg and 3 cun above the most prominent point of the medial malleolus (large inner ankle bone). Especially in women,
there is often a palpable depression in that area.

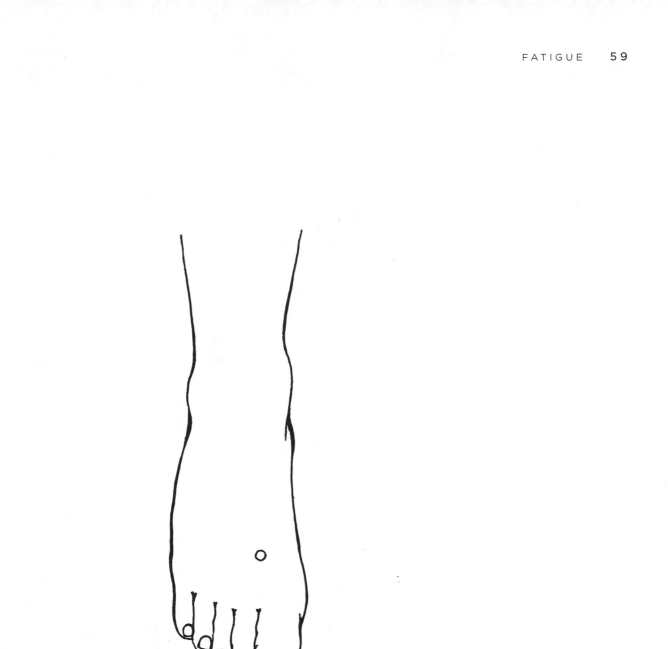

LV3 (Liver Channel)

This point can be found on the top of the foot between the first and second toes at the proximal point where the body and base regions of both metatarsal bones meet.

Smell: Herbs, Flowers, Plants, and Essential Oils*— Lemon and Rosemary

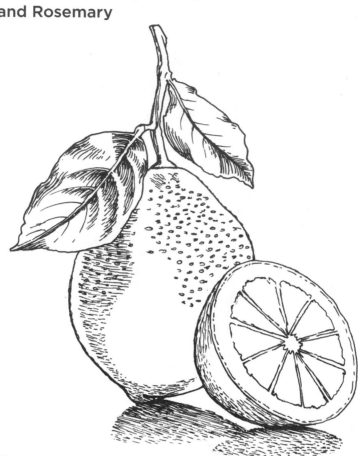

Lemon

This fruit is believed to have originated in India. Its medicinal and therapeutic qualities are many. Today, lemons are cultivated in China and Mexico. Used in aromatherapy, lemon oil is known for its calming qualities and pleasant aroma. It is often mixed with other oils whose aromas may be unattractive or overpowering for some people. It's reputed to have a mood-lifting effect on people, thus countering the low energy of fatigue. The Japanese have been known to diffuse lemon oil through the ventilation systems of their offices because of its ability to increase attention and concentration.

*Essential Oils (EO) have several methods of use. Please refer to the Treatment Protocol Information and Resource Guide of this book (page 197) for additional detailed information on aromatherapy.

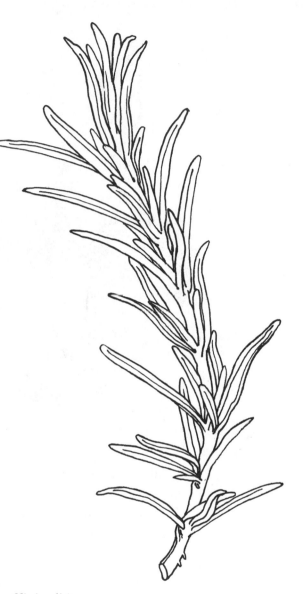

Rosemary (*Rosmarinus officinalis*)

Native to southern Europe, rosemary is also reputed to help memory, so much so that in contemporary Greece students getting ready for tests will burn some rosemary the night before to improve their performance. In ancient Greece, students made garlands of rosemary for the same purpose. In cooking, rosemary (part of the mint family of plants) adds a spark to many beloved Mediterranean dishes. Inhaling rosemary is a very natural and safe pick-me-up for the brain.

Taste: Herbal Tisanes*—Basil, Ginkgo

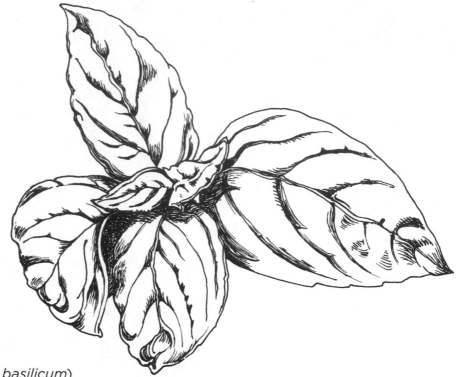

Basil (*Ocimum basilicum*)

Basil originated in India and spread relatively recently to Europe around the sixteenth century. It is generally useful in reducing stress and anxiety, which are often contributing factors in fatigue. Used in aromatherapy with other herbs like peppermint, basil has been seen to improve mental focus for people who feel acute mental fatigue. It can also be prepared as an herbal tisane beverage. In ancient Indian (Ayurvedic) medicine, basil is considered one of the holiest and most sacred herbs. So sacred in fact, that it is often planted around temples to serve as a protector. According to modern medicine, some preliminary studies have associated basil with improving mental focus, alertness, and attention. One study combined it with other essential oils—peppermint and helichrysum—and found a beneficial effect on exhaustion. (Varney & Buckle, 2013)

*Tea and herbal tisanes are easy to prepare and find at local stores and markets. For detailed information on preparation and sourcing please refer to the Treatment Protocol Information and Resource Guide on page 197.

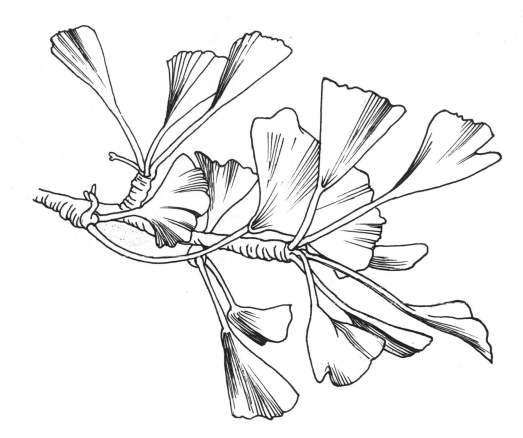

Ginkgo (*Ginkgo biloba*)

Ginkgo is an ancient plant that has been found in fossil remains dating back about 270 million years. It has been used in traditional Chinese medicine for centuries. The extracts from the plant can increase blood flow to the brain, thus helping to revive people who are experiencing fatigue or low energy. (Cieza et al., 2003)

Sight: Yoga Postures—Downward-Facing Dog, Big Toe Pose, Cobra Pose

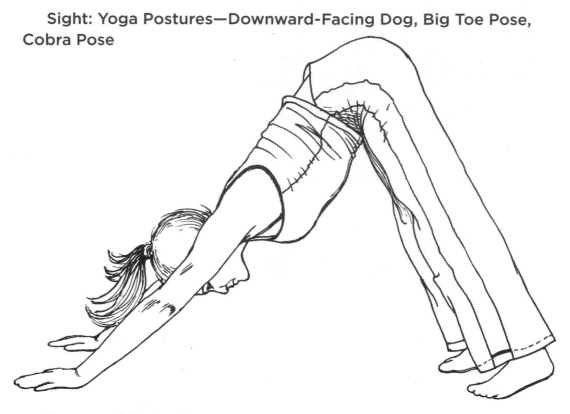

Downward-Facing Dog

This may be the best-known pose in yoga. Why? First, it's probably the yoga pose that most closely resembles its name. When you do this one, you look like a puppy stretching out to meet his master. While it looks playful, it can be challenging as it engages the whole body pretty vigorously. While balance is minimally challenged if the pose is done correctly, the legs and hamstrings are fully engaged and the head is upside down, balancing between the arms. To get into this pose, begin by kneeling on the floor. Facing forward, get on all fours and try your best to get your body in a straight line, aligning hands with shoulders and with hips. With arms extended, lift your pelvis upward. For beginners, this quickly becomes a strenuous pose, so be gentle with yourself. To deepen the pose, you can push your heels toward the ground and gently push your fingers forward (Rea, 2007b). Like many poses known as inversions, Downward Dog promises benefits in diminishing fatigue. Inversions are supposed to help support the immune and endocrine systems. It also allows blood to flow to the brain easily and can revive the lower body and legs if they are not receiving enough blood due to any circulation problems.

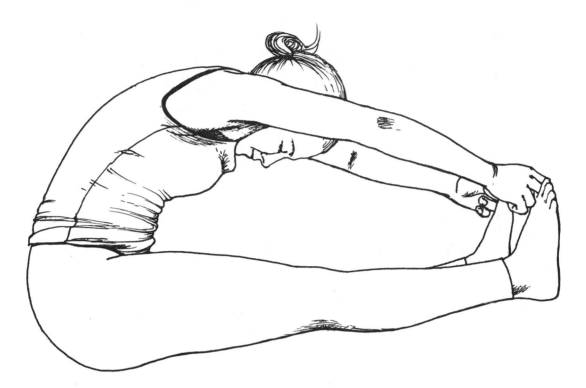

Big Toe Pose

This pose gets its name from the fact that it's held in place while you are bending over and holding your big toes. If you can't reach your toes, bend over as much as you can and maintain the pose by holding a strap that is wrapped around the balls of the feet. Try to press your toes into your hand (or pull gently on the straps). As you breathe, lift your chest and stretch your arms with an inhale and then release your chest and bend toward your toes with an exhale (Big Toe Pose, 2015).

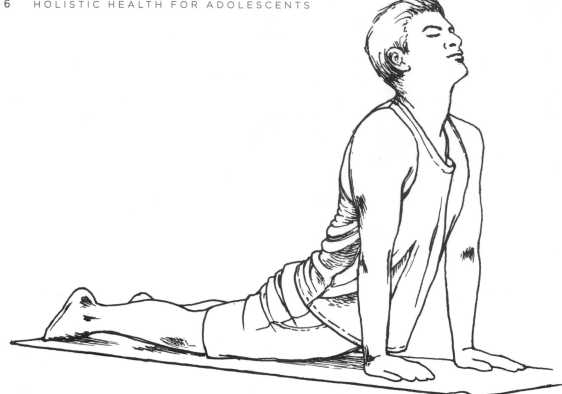

Cobra Pose

Some of the benefits of the back bend called Cobra include strengthening the entire back while improving its flexibility. It also tones thighs and buttocks. It opens the chest, which is not too common in everyday movement. Doing this can release tensions in the chest that are often overlooked, thus perhaps gently releasing some pent-up emotions and letting good feelings enter the body. The pose begins with lying on the floor. The key preparation for the movement involves putting your hands underneath your shoulders. Then pull your shoulder blades back and place your elbows close to your body. Engage your legs and then lift the chest while making sure that your thighs keep contact with the ground. Aim to open the chest rather than trying to lift the head as high as possible (Rea, 2007a). This pose alleviates fatigue by improving blood circulation and promoting better breathing through opening the chest.

Sound: Steady Sounds and Upbeat, Positive Music

Music therapists have found that often the most effective music is that which is already familiar to the listener. Steady, upbeat, and positive-sounding music is combined with other stimuli to decrease the fatigue (real or perceived) of patients. In some cases, guided imagery can be combined with music to improve patients' feelings of well-being. In cases involving physical fatigue (as in physical or occupational therapy settings), music can be aligned with exercises and has been seen as a positive distraction from feelings of fatigue in patients (Lim, Miller, & Fabian, 2011).

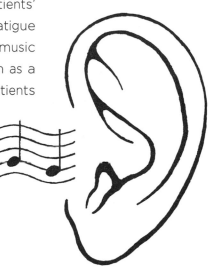

CHAPTER 4

Low Mood

/////////////////////////

DANNY'S PROBLEM WITH LOW MOOD

Some kids need help with their mental and emotional well-being because they're high achievers, trying to fit as many activities as they can into a day. That was the case with Carlos and his persistent fatigue, as we just saw in Chapter 3. But, as with adults, even more of my patients feel tense and pressured because they are thrust into high-stakes and stressful situations that push their capacities to the breaking point. Such was the case with Danny, a boy of 17 who came to the school clinic suffering from low mood.

When Danny came into my clinic, he was dealing with a wide array of problems that had moved him into a low mood. His father, a widower, was concerned and brought Danny in after hearing about the clinic. Danny's low mood had persisted for a while. His father was wondering if he might need medication, but was hoping to find alternatives. While there was no history of depression in his family, Danny was facing a number of very difficult situations that really tested his resiliency.

Major changes were happening in Danny's home. His mother had passed away from a sudden illness 2 years before. Besides the general hardship of losing a parent, the loss of Danny's mother had other major impacts on him and his family. The loss of her income created financial pressure. As the oldest of four children, Danny lept into that financial void by getting a weekend job (which wasn't easy to find). Then, about 6 months before Danny first came to the clinic, his dad lost his job. Danny felt that it was his duty to set an example for his siblings and tried to put a brave face on this difficult situation for them, which put even more pressure on him.

A partial solution arose when his dad, a construction worker, got a chance at a 6-month job in Connecticut. While this would help to mend the family finances, the temporary nature of the job and the financial climate made it very difficult for him to move his family to the adjoining state. Danny's aunts and uncles would help take care of the kids, but they weren't sure if the four siblings would stay in their apartment or be split up among family members in the area. In addition, Danny was looking ahead: He was hoping to go to a local community college but didn't know if that would be feasible for the family. All this change and responsibility kept him from participating in typical teenage social activities, such as after-school clubs, sports, or just spending time with friends. He was a naturally athletic kid and especially wanted to participate in some sort of sports team. He felt that his life choices were being curtailed in a significant way.

Luckily, Danny was open to finding ways to help himself feel better. One major reason for this was that one of his friends had recently received acupuncture, an integrative treatment that seemed to have worked.

LOW MOOD: WHAT IS IT?

Low mood is a minor form of depression. The two conditions share many of the same symptoms. Symptoms of low mood and depression are very similar, but low mood can be dealt with more easily and turned back relatively quickly with the appropriate interventions. Depression occurs when low mood is deeply established in a person's life and emotions, thus becoming more a habit of mind than a short-term condition. A child who is suffering from depression needs more help than he or she can find at my clinics. But preventative measures drawn from integrative medicine can stop many cases of low mood from spiraling down into depression.

Symptoms of low mood can often signal depression. While an individual's low mood might improve if issues or concerns are resolved, some types of depression can often last longer and may require more conventional types of treatment, including psychopharmaceuticals and psychotherapy. One researcher explains the small but very important difference between low mood and depression: "Low mood describes a temporary emotional and physiological state in humans, typically characterized by fatigue, loss of motivation and interest, anhedonia (loss of pleasure in previously pleasurable activities), pessimism about future actions, locomotor retardation and other symptoms such as crying. . . . When low mood is extreme or prolonged, it is designated clinical depression" (Nettle, 2008). Adults need to pay attention to their kids' moods so that what starts out as a low-mood phase does not turn into a more lasting state of being.

Parents should also guard against their own prejudices concerning mental health. Unfortunately, many people think depression only affects adults, but children and adolescents can also succumb to this impairment. As many as two-thirds of people with depression do not realize they have a treatable illness and therefore do not seek professional help (Halverson, 2015). If adults ignore their children's signs of depression, the kids will be even less likely to see it in themselves. Predictably, rates of undertreatment for depression are higher among teens than adults (Thapar, Collishaw, Potter, & Thapar, 2010).

For parents, distinguishing between normal ups and downs and a more serious emotional health problem in children or adolescents is not always an easy thing to do. When a child is not able to function at school and has lost interest in things that were important to him or her, such as being part of a sports team or attending after-school events, low mood is probably the problem. Parents should address this as soon as possible by talking with children about what is troubling them. While a child's low mood may not present itself as a big problem for parents, it might be a major problem for the child.

While integrative treatments can help with depression, depressive disorders are too severe for integrative treatments alone. Because low mood and depression can be confused with one another, it's important to be aware of different kinds of depression that are not low mood.

Classifications of depression include major depressive disorder (MDD), a common psychiatric disorder characterized by persistent low mood and impaired social function (Cai, 2015); depression with melancholic features; atypical depression (like normal depression except more responsive to positive events); psychotic features; bipolar depression; unipolar depression disorder (UDD); and seasonal affective disorder (SAD). In adolescence, UDD is often unrecognized and the incidence, especially in girls, rises sharply after puberty (Thapar, 2010).

The question of why low mood and depression exist in the first place has caught the attention of researchers, mainly because depression seems so unhealthy and unproductive for our species. But by imagining how low-mood symptoms may have first evolved in the context of small villages and similar places where humans first lived in groups, one can see how low mood could actually help individuals adapt to adverse situations. For instance, self-reproach is a common symptom of low mood. Doubting and questioning ourselves, now as well as in the past, can help us examine how we may have contributed to an accident or a problem. From an evolutionary standpoint, self-reproach may have helped individuals to survive in a tribe or village because signaling "culpability to others [would help] to avoid the loss of important social bonds." Similarly, sleeplessness derived from low mood may have also helped early humans. "Nocturnal wakefulness," a researcher writes, "could protect against attacks by animals or humans. Although modern life has become relatively safe, dangers from predators were very real for our ancestors." In some cases, depression in the modern day can be seen as a product of evolutionary behaviors that no longer correspond to the environment. Unfortunately for many humans, the pace and scale of change in the modern world often outpace the speed of our evolutionary adaptations (Keller & Nesse, 2005).

CAUSES OF LOW MOOD

There is no single formula that can predict whether or not an adolescent may drift into low mood or depression. However, three contributing factors often combine to make particular adolescents more susceptible than the norm.

Temporal and Situational Influences

Kids moving into their teen years are facing an incredible amount of change with very little experience to draw upon. As mentioned earlier, people generally feel less stress as they get older, probably due to lessons from life experience. Adolescents, on the other hand, don't yet have these lessons as they enter puberty. As their bodies and brain change at unprecedented rates, they also are put into more complex social situations. They are beginning to become sexually mature and questions concerning relations (both social and sexual) with the opposite sex can become both very important and very mysterious, contributing to the feeling of sometimes overwhelming change in their lives. Finally, just as in adults, major life changes (such as a move or a death in the family) can provoke low mood. Teenagers' lack of experience with these kinds of problems may make their recovery from such changes more difficult.

Familial and Genetic Influences

Studies have found that depression does tend to be familial. These family influences are both behavioral and, potentially, genetic. In general, teens whose parents have suffered depression are three to four times more likely than other teens to feel depression themselves (Thapar et al., 2010). One obvious influence is a child witnessing one of his parents going through depression. This not only saddens or worries the child but also sets an example of a (poor) coping strategy to deal with difficult situations. Whether or not this influence is also genetic as well as behavioral has been harder to determine (Rice, Harold, & Thapar, 2002).

Changes in the Brain

Throughout a human being's lifetime, the brain has a wonderful characteristic—plasticity. It can grow and adapt throughout life. During adolescence, the brain is particularly plastic. This has two implications. First, it means that kids have a tremendous capacity to learn and change in positive ways. Second, that openness leaves them susceptible to negative or damaging influences. Certainly, drugs such as alcohol or marijuana have a much bigger impact (i.e., addictive potential) on adolescents compared to adults because a kid's brain is much more open to integrating the chemicals from those drugs into its systems. An episode of binge drinking, for instance, has a much more severe impact (e.g., memory loss) than it would for an adult (Jensen & Nutt, 2015). Moreover, it's been observed that teens with deeply emotionally involving relationships during high school often underperform academically and can have more emotional difficulty in later years.

It's become a bit of a truism in the psychological professions that one thing that distinguishes teens from adults is the development of their prefrontal cortex in the brain. This is where many of the regulatory functions of human behavior are developed: shaping memory, organizational capacities, planning for the future, and controlling mood. It was once thought that this part of the brain would develop completely in childhood, but scientists were surprised to find that so much of this part of the brain was still growing and developing through adolescence. How exactly this phenomenon translates into low mood or depression is hard to say. Certainly, a developed frontal cortex is no guarantee against bad judgment in adult years. However, underdevelopment may explain teens' tendency to indulge in risky and unwise behavior, which can certainly contribute to low mood and depression when taking uncalculated risks turn out badly (Spink, 2002).

LOW MOOD AND THE ADOLESCENT POPULATION

Depression in adolescents appears highest in low-income and middle-income countries, and is associated with many present and future health problems, as well as a heightened suicide risk (Thapar, 2012). In the United States, around 11% of adolescents have some form of depressive disorder by age 18 (National Institute of Mental Health, 2015b). According to data gathered in 2012, the rate of depression is low at the end of the preteen years (3.7%) and climbs quickly by the time kids reach age 15 or 16 (11.8%). It then begins to come down (perhaps with the benefit of a little more experience?), with 10.9% of U.S. teens reporting the occurrence of a major depressive episode (National Institute of Mental Health, 2015c).

Physiology of Low Mood and Depression

Major depressive disorder is characterized by persistent low mood and impaired social function. Recent scientific evidence identified the involvement of neurotrophic factors, inflammatory cytokines, the hypothalamus-pituitary-adrenal axis, and glutamate receptors in the pathophysiology of this illness. Researchers report that integration of the MDD-related signal pathways causes brain-derived neurotrophic factor dysfunction and increased cell death (Cai 2015). This factor is a protein found in the brain and spinal cord that promotes neuronal (nerve cell) survival when functioning optimally. The neurotransmitter serotonin is also implicated in MDD. Serotonin is involved in the regulation of many brain functions, including appetite, mood, sexual behavior, sleep, and even our fear response. The role of central nervous system serotonin activity in the pathophysiology of MDD is suggested by the therapeutic efficacy of selective serotonin reuptake inhibitors (Halverson, 2015).

Signs and Symptoms

There are obvious red flags that signal low mood in adolescence:

- Reduced school or professional performance
- Withdrawal from friends and activities
- Aggressive, violent behavior
- Repeat consultations for ill-defined complaints
- Family conflict
- Difficulty sleeping or concentrating
- Lethargy
- Apathy
- Changes in eating habits
- Poor motivation and concentration
- Feelings of low self-esteem and worthlessness
- Irritability (more prominent in adolescents than in adults)

The Anxiety and Depression Association of America cautions that if an adolescent's symptoms last for more than 2 weeks and interfere with regular daily activities and family and school, then the child may have a depressive disorder. It is important to note that an enduring low mood may persist despite some deceptive signs that the adolescent is functioning normally. What compounds the difficulty in realizing that low mood is a problem for a child is that young people can successfully compartmentalize their low mood symptoms. A child suffering from low mood may be able to maintain normal functioning in some components of life (such as socializing or maintaining athletic activities) while performing poorly in others (such as academic work or family life; Roberts, 2013).

Low mood often presents with irritability and disruptive behavioral disorders and is fairly common in the 11- to 19-year-old group (Roberts, 2013). Internationally accepted diagnostic criteria for depression in adolescents are considered to be the same as for adults; however, irritability is a more prominent feature in adolescents, as is frequency of comorbidity of psychological problems (Thapar et al., 2010). Because of these features in adolescents, diagnosis of low mood or depression is challenging for physicians, mainly due to the unique developmental changes that occur during the adolescent years.

BAD COPING MECHANISMS FOR DEPRESSION

More than the other mental health issues discussed in this book, low mood is closely associated with an individual's thoughts. In the absence of professional health care, adolescents suffering from low mood often reinforce their feelings by adopting negative thinking patterns that explain or make sense of the difficult situations in which they find themselves. These includes thinking patterns such as catastrophizing (predicting the worst possible outcome), mind reading (believing other people perceive them negatively), and bias against themselves (overlooking their strengths and overemphasizing their weaknesses; Williams & Garland, 2002). When an adolescent exhibits thinking patterns such as these, low mood or depression is definitely a possible cause.

Some behaviors that tend to be associated with low mood are also contrasting but related. At one extreme, people with low mood may try to cope by withdrawing from socializing and other situations that might provoke feelings of unhappiness or inadequacy. Similarly, they may also repress the expression of their feelings in order not to draw attention to themselves. At the opposite extreme, teens may unexpectedly express their repressed feelings by lashing out at those around them or by general irritability.

TREATMENT PROTOCOLS AND SUPPORTIVE THERAPIES

The holistic approach to treating depression in young people focuses on treating the whole being, body and mind. Often meditation is used in combination with conventional medicine.

Across most patient populations, the combination of medication and psychotherapy generally provides the quickest and most sustained response for treatment of depression (Ishak, 2011); however, the Anxiety and Depression Association of America reports that there is a growing body of scientific evidence about the benefits of complementary and alternative medicine (CAM) treatment, which is not conventional medical treatment but is used in conjunction with conventional medicine. Currently, the following CAM practices are used to treat anxiety and depressive disorders (Anxiety and Depression Association of America, 2015).

CAM Relaxation Techniques to Counter Low Mood and Depression

Yoga and Meditation

Yoga is a holistic practice that emphasizes mind-body connectedness and involves postures, breathing, and meditation. Today there is a growing recognition by scientists and health professionals that yoga promotes physical and mental well-being. The physical benefits of yoga include improved flexibility, strength, and posture. Some of the many psychological benefits include stress reduction, increased self-awareness, inner peace and calm, increased energy and vitality, increased mental clarity, improved reaction time, improved sleep, and increased emotional stability (McCall, 2007). Adolescents should be encouraged to experiment to find the yoga postures that best suit their body and temperament. When they discover how a physical activity can have a strong and helpful impact on the state of their mind, young yoga practitioners often develop true enthusiasm that then accelerates the improvement of their mood.

Acupuncture

In traditional Chinese belief, depression is a problem with poor qi circulation around the body and affecting specific organs (liver, heart, and spleen). Acupuncture treatment increases the flow of qi, stimulating source points on both hands between the thumb and index finger and both feet between the big toe and the second toe is one example (Errington-Evans, 2011; Ljubinovic, 2015; Eshkevari et al., 2013). While the exact corporeal mechanisms behind acupuncture are difficult to determine, some animal experiments have shown a direct correlation between, for instance, acupuncture and reduced stress (Eshkevari et al., 2013).

Herbs and Vitamins

Studies in adults and children have found that folate, vitamin B_{12}, and zinc levels are lower in depressed than nondepressed persons. It has been found that supplementing with these vitamins and minerals can lead to improvements in mood (Sawi & Breuner, 2012).

Massage Therapy

Some research concludes that massage therapy is significant in alleviating symptoms of depression (Hou, Chiang, Hsu, Chiu, & Yen, 2010). Thirty minutes of daily massage therapy administered to depressed adolescents resulted in improvement in mood and behavior (Moyer, Rounds, & Hannum, 2004).

Art, Music, or Dance Therapy

Art therapies can be very important CAM approaches to decrease depression and increase vitality (Koch, Morlinghaus, & Fuch, 2007). These therapies are gaining acceptance as they help facilitate psychologic adjustment, and provide an alternate platform of self-expression. These therapies are also of benefit to expand treatment options as they can be blended or added to other treatment modalities with relative ease.

Food and Nutrition

Unhealthy foods—especially sugary ones—are easy to access and may boost mood for a short time, but after a few hours energy level will drop and an unpleasant feeling may reappear. Eating a healthy diet rich in vegetables, beans, whole grains, fruits, fish, and lean meats will provide a lot more energy and boost mood, which is very important for depression. Eight steps to eat right for depression include the following (Greenlaw, 2010):

1. *Share a meal:* having a friend or family member with you may improve your mood.
2. *Choose food wisely:* Eat a healthy diet.
3. *Avoid alcohol:* Alcohol is a depressant and may worsen depression.
4. *Eliminate added sugar and caffeine from diet:* Sugar and caffeine can cause blood sugar to rise and fall during day, leading to mood swings.
5. *Supplement your diet:* Some nutrients such as omega-3 fatty acids are found

in salmon, albacore tuna, tofu, soybeans, and walnuts. Folate is found in beans, green vegetables, and orange juice. Vitamin B$_{12}$ is found in meats, fish, milk, and eggs.

6. *Keep a journal:* Record everything eaten or drunk during a day and track moods. Different foods and combinations of foods affect people differently.
7. *Eat regular meals:* Maintaining regular meals will keep blood sugar stable and prevent mood swings.
8. *Healthy snacks:* Fruits, nuts, yogurt, carrot sticks, hummus, and whole-wheat crackers are wonderful between-meal snacks.

Exercise

Regular exercise and activity produces a positive effect on mood and energy level. Also, research has shown that exercise causes biochemical changes in the brain that are similar to those produced by medication, including an increase in serotonin levels (Blumenthal et al., 2007).

Education

Parental involvement in treating depression in adolescence is very important to achieving success. Adolescents as well as their parents need to gain an understanding of how depression can affect a child's mood, thoughts, body, and behavior. This is accomplished through education (Moreland & Bonin, 2015):

- Understanding of symptoms of depression and how they impact relationships
- Recognition of recurring symptoms
- Ways to help the adolescent with depression

HELPING DANNY

At our first meeting I could tell Danny was on the fence about the usefulness of alternative treatments. Let's face it, aromatherapy was not in a young man's vocabulary, and consequently, Danny saw the interventions as "anything but a guy thing." So my first objective was to legitimize the treatments by, for example, explaining the World Health Organization's endorsement of acupuncture as a treatment for more than 40 medical conditions. I also mentioned that elite athletes use acupressure, acupuncture, and trigger point therapy to enhance their performance and calm the mind. He soon realized that these noninvasive measures had merit, and I won Danny's buy-in.

During the first several weeks of his treatment, Danny would come in once a week and we would focus on helping him reduce his stress. I started with some simple approaches. He tried using some acupressure points as well as aromatherapy, especially essential oils that were citrus based, such as grapefruit or orange, that he found uplifting. When he felt badly, he would try an acupressure point or open a towelette that I had infused with oil for aromatherapy.

After these approaches began to work, he then asked for more options that would help with low mood throughout the day; he was open to yoga and physical interventions because he was an active kid. So he started to use certain yoga positions that he would do when he had a free moment in the afternoon in addition to acupressure when he went to sleep at night. The yoga at home was so helpful that he soon became involved in a local yoga program for teens, which he found very beneficial. For adolescents, whose bodies are going through almost explosive growth, it's important to choose yoga positions that avoid hyperextension. I introduce yoga positions from books, or from photos and videos online.

Then, something gratifying for me happened: He began to internalize these treatments and make them his own. He started to figure out the specific things that worked for him when, where, and how he needed them. His preferences included acupressure points and certain yoga positions, as well as meditative techniques using music while holding a specific yoga position, such as a forward bend. He essentially transformed his learning into a personalized treatment plan. Over time his "downs" or low moods, as he described them, became less severe and decreased in duration. From that point on, he felt that he was more able to actively engage in treatments to counteract negative feelings. Within about 2 weeks, Danny developed a sense of mastery and control over his state of mind. No longer would an emotional trigger (such as the recurrent feeling that he didn't have enough friends) inevitably lead to a downward spiral, affecting his mood for the rest of the day. He always had something in his toolbox that he could employ to counteract what was going on.

It was a wonderful thing to watch how Danny was starting to get control over his low mood by becoming the mastermind of his personalized treatment protocol. When he completed treatment at the clinic, he reported in a questionnaire that he was feeling much better and that he was happy that he had the tools he needed to help himself in the future.

CHAPTER 4 LOW MOOD SENSORY TREATMENT PROTOCOL*

Touch: Acupressure Points**—LV3, PC6, ST41

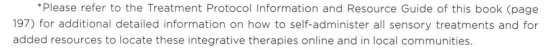

LV3 (Liver Channel)

This acupuncture point can be found on the top of the foot between the first and second toes at the proximal point where the body and base regions of both metatarsal bones meet.

*Please refer to the Treatment Protocol Information and Resource Guide of this book (page 197) for additional detailed information on how to self-administer all sensory treatments and for added resources to locate these integrative therapies online and in local communities.

**For all acupressure points: Once you locate the point, stimulate it by pressing down with your index or middle finger and provide moderate pressure. Rotate your finger in a circular motion while pressing over the point. Continue to stimulate or massage the area for 2–3 minutes. Can be repeated as needed.

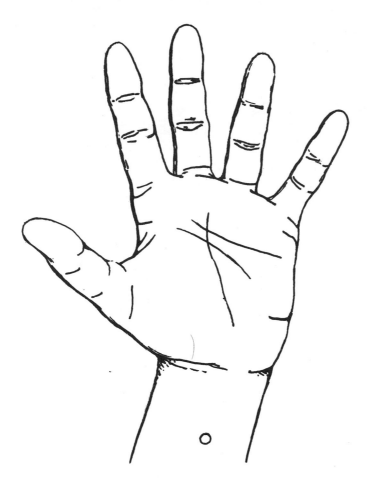

PC6

This point is located on the pericardium (PC) channel. It can be found approximately 2 cun from the crease of the wrist. Acupoints on the limbs (arms and legs) are bilateral. So while they may be shown on one side of the body, they are intended for bilateral application.

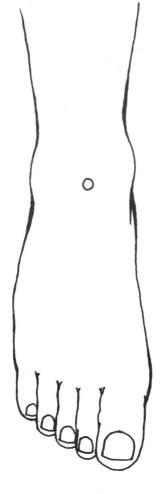

ST41 (Stomach Channel)

This point sits on the front of the foot, located at the midpoint of the transverse crease of the ankle joint, in the depression between two tendons: the tendons of muscle extensor digitorum longus and hallucis longus, approximately at the level of the tip of the external ankle joint.

Smell: Herbs, Flowers, Plants, and Essential Oils*—Bergamot, Clary Sage, Tangerine

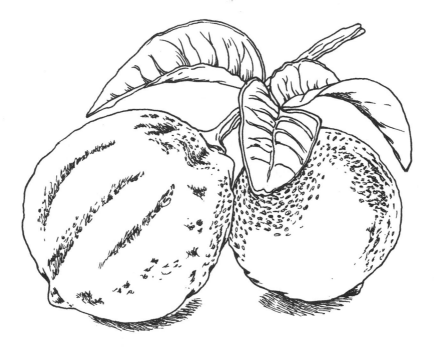

Bergamot (*Citrus bergamia*)

This is a fruit from an evergreen tree, originating in Asia, that is now cultivated principally in southern Italy. It's likely that the name comes from the Italian town of Bergamo, where it was first grown commercially. It is widely used as a flavoring in Earl Grey tea. Its principal use in aromatherapy is as an antidepressant, and it also reduces tension. Its citrus qualities help to counter volatile emotions like anger and irritability. It also helps to release tension and pent-up emotions leading to low mood by helping people relax.

*Essential Oils (EO) have several methods of use. Please refer to the Treatment Protocol Information and Resource Guide of this book (page 197) for additional detailed information on aromatherapy.

Clary Sage (*Salvia sclarea*)

This herb is related to garden sage. Although both can be used in aroma-therapy, common sage (*Salvia officinalis*) sometimes can cause unwanted side effects. The name Clary is derived from the Latin word for "clear," which is *clarus*. This evokes its historical ability to improve vision as well as ameliorate tired or overstrained eyes. It has a calming quality that can alleviate stress or insomnia that can contribute to low mood.

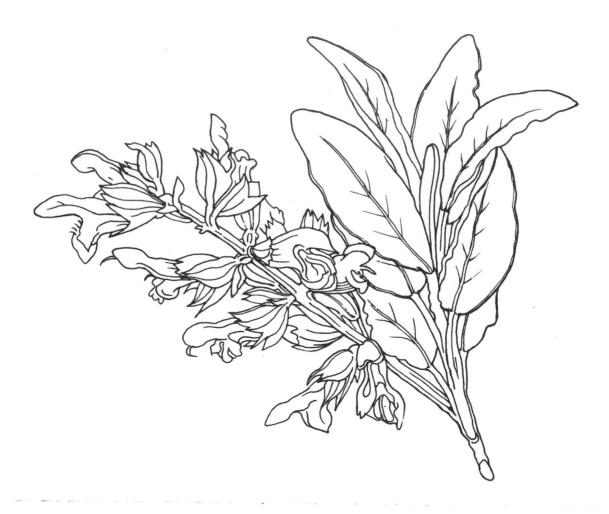

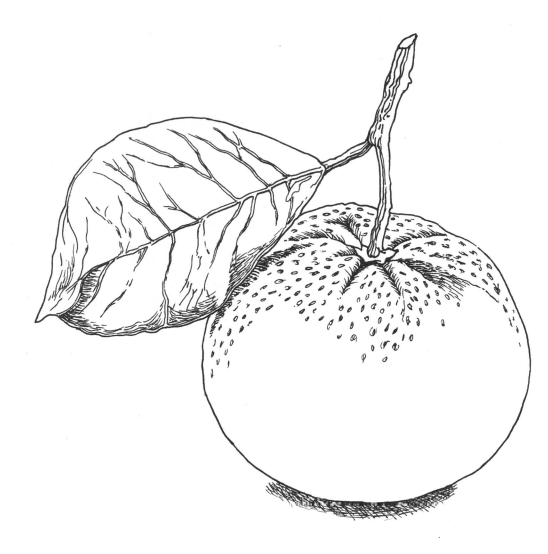

Tangerine (*Citrus tangerina*)

For low mood, the citrus fruit tangerine can have an uplifting effect on emotions. Native to Southeast Asia, this fruit has a fresh sweet scent that can be both reviving and refreshing. Tangerine essential oil contains limonene, which is known for its antioxidant activity. (Komori, et al., 1995)

Taste: Herbal Tisanes*—Saffron and Ginkgo

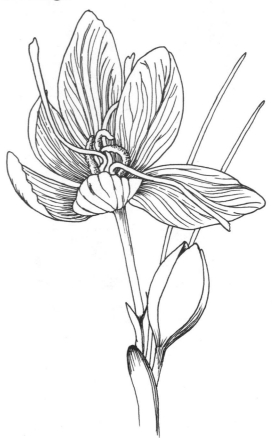

Saffron (*Crocus sativus*)

Saffon comes from the saffron crocus flower. It is not derived from the purple flower of the crocus, but rather the dried stigmas of the flower. (Stigmas are found within the flower and catch pollen.) Saffron is very expensive, perhaps the most expensive spice around because about one pound of saffron takes 250,000 stigmas. Good thing that it's pretty powerful and is usually used in very small amounts. It is a good treatment for low mood or mild depression. One study showed a significant reduction in depression from taking saffron in capsule form for 6 weeks compared to placebo (Akhondzade et al., 2005). Saffron can be incorporated into many recipes, making it easy to consume.

*Tea and herbal tisanes are easy to prepare and find at local stores and markets. For detailed information on preparation and sourcing please refer to the Treatment Protocol Information and Resource Guide on page 197.

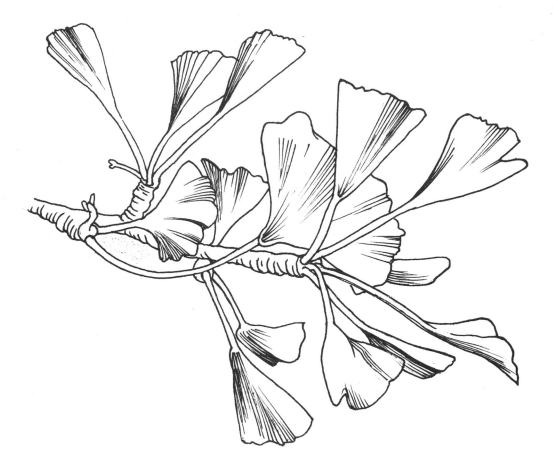

Ginkgo (*Ginkgo biloba*)

As mentioned earlier, ginkgo is an ancient plant that has been used for centuries in traditional Chinese medicine. The extracts from the plant have been associated with increased blood flow to the brain, which can help reduce fatigue. Some studies have highlighted a similar impact on the nervous system and found ginkgo to not only support cerebral blood flow but also aid in focus and attentional difficulties. One of the causes of depression can be traced to low serotonin levels in the brain. Ginkgo can aid in the increase of serotonin levels and act as an ameliorative to restoring optimal brain function. (Cieza et al., 2003; Salehi et al., 2003)

Sight: Yoga Postures— Fish Pose, Legs Up Wall, Downward-Facing Dog

Fish Pose

If you can do this pose in the water, so the story goes, you can float. The pose is performed lying down, face up, so you may look more like a fish floundering out of water. No matter what you may think you look like, Fish Pose has great benefits. Like Cobra Pose, the hands are pulled in close to the body, this time below the buttocks. Elbows are also tucked in. When you inhale, combine two movements that are mutually reinforcing: Lift the chest while you allow your head to rest on the floor. (It's important to combine the two because it's hard to lift the chest while also supporting your head.) But don't have your head support its own weight too much; this will prevent you from overstressing your neck.

Legs Up Wall

This is a passive pose that is probably harder to get into than maintain. It's like sitting in a chair that's tipped back onto the floor. The key choice to make in this case is whether or not to use a support or a bolster. For those who feel like their lower back might be strained with their legs lying perpendicularly, some sort of bolster to support the back can be very helpful. To start, sit next to a wall with your left side pressing against the wall; then, lie back and lift your legs up against the wall, moving your buttocks toward the wall as well. Shift the weight in your legs and buttocks until you're comfortable. Hold this for 5 or 10 minutes, breathing normally but with an awareness of your breath. This calming and relaxing pose can relieve feelings of anxiety and offers potential help for those dealing with low mood.

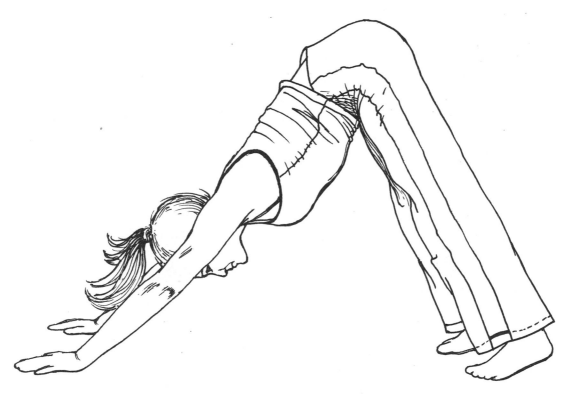

Downward-Facing Dog

Because this pose is an inversion—placing the head below the heart—it can help relax the nervous system. The calming nature of the pose helps to balance the often overworked minds of people undergoing depression. And looking at the world upside down does give you the chance of getting a fresh perspective.

Sound: Energizing Music, Upbeat Tempos, Uplifting Sounds

For people experiencing low mood or depression, it has been found that participating in making music can be very helpful. While the reasons for this are unclear, one theory is that playing music may be effective because "active music-making within the therapeutic frame offers the patient opportunities for new aesthetic, physical and relational experiences" (Maratos, 2011). Energizing music, upbeat tempos, and uplifting sounds and lyrics are the most helpful elements for people experiencing low mood.

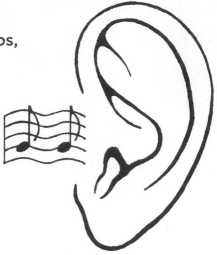

One could even try clapping along to familiar and unfamiliar music to boost energy and alertness. This allows people to express themselves in nonverbal ways, which is helpful for people struggling to articulate the problems lying behind low mood and depression. And for adolescents who may be particularly reluctant to deal with their depression in a therapeutic setting, music may also be a much less threatening intervention (Maratos, Crawford, & Procter, 2011; Parker-Hope, 2008).

CHAPTER 5

Sleep Difficulty

///

CAROLINA'S TROUBLE WITH SLEEPING

When Carolina came to my clinic, she was suffering from the common problems of being overtaxed and overstressed, with too many things on her mind. Her chief complaint was having difficulty both falling asleep at night and staying asleep. She was a quiet eleventh grader. She was long, lean, and strong—a natural athlete. But her drooping eyes and dragging feet were signs of some real problems. She was very stressed about being a junior in high school. She was hoping to be the first in her family to go to college, and felt that she couldn't risk letting that opportunity slip through her hands. At school, she often didn't feel very well accepted socially. She was also working after school to help with finances. Finally, she had to help raise some of her younger siblings to help her mom, who was single.

She had a lot of different responsibilities to fulfill; many issues connected to these responsibilities would bother her at night and she would start obsessing. Her sleep suffered terribly. This would lead to more problems, like getting to school late, falling asleep in class, or not having the energy to do things. She was just dragging because she couldn't get things done at night.

A phenomenon that plagues teens all over the world is difficulty getting enough sleep. Many parents have witnessed their bleary-eyed teens looking half-dead over breakfast, complaining about having to go to school so early. The number of hours kids sleep gets cut down for a lot of reasons—some predictable, and some new. An early school start time chips away at a teen's sleep schedule. Simultaneously, adolescents' inner clocks have them falling asleep later in the evening. This age-old problem can be exacerbated by teens communicating late at night via modern gadgets like cell phones and iPads.

Luckily, Carolina wasn't too involved in modern gadgetry and expressed an interest in learning techniques to get to sleep in a natural way. She was also ready to commit to changing her sleep habits—not something that comes easily to teens. As any parent knows, trying to pressure your teenager to fall sleep earlier is often a fruitless campaign. Good sleep habits usually emerge from teens' own initiatives.

Often must I appeal to my clients' self-image by explaining the connection between good sleep and radiant skin. During sleep, hormones and antioxidants are released that actually promote regenerative bodily processes and help the skin's natural healing process, which supports a good complexion. This realization often has a powerful effect on teens and gets them on board to establish better sleep awareness. But Carolina didn't have any reluctance to commit to an earlier bedtime. The challenge was finding a way to get her to fall asleep earlier, and then stay asleep.

THE IMPORTANCE AND MYSTERY OF SLEEP

What is sleep? Why do we sleep? And what does sleep really do? These questions may not occur to us often because sleep is such a fundamental part of our being that we just take it as a given: We assume sleep functions to rest a living organism after activity. But once we examine sleep and try to ask detailed and probing questions of this phenomenon, we find that answers about it are not so easy to find.

The scientific debates that swirl around the topic of sleep are far from resolved, but nobody doubts that sleep is supremely important to human mental and physical health. One indication of sleep's role in optimal human functioning is suggested by how active the brain is during sleep. According to one scientist, "The amplitude of the changes in brain metabolism and neuronal activity that occurs during sleep exceeds those which occur during most waking periods" (Siegel, 2005). Indeed, while humans are passive in the world during sleep, their bodies and brains get a lot of important work done.

Traditionally, many scientists assumed that sleep was evolutionarily maladaptive, because there were so many other things human beings could be doing to promote the survival of the species: hunting, mating, eating, cultivating food, and building shelter and defenses, among other productive activities. With this line of reasoning, it seemed natural to deduce that what was going on in the brain and body during sleep had to be even more important.

However, there are other ways of looking at sleep that don't depict sleep as competing with other important functions. In other words, more recent research suggests inductively that there is no zero-sum game between sleep and other important human activities and that sleep is quite adaptive to evolutionary needs. Indeed, the more we see sleep as a passive response to environmental stimuli as well as an active tool of evolutionary adaptation, the easier it is to understand. (In this way, sleep resembles the way the senses, as described earlier in this book, are the result of interactions between the internal and the external, between the brain and the outside stimuli gathered through the body.)

While sleep can be synonymous with rest, it is not accurately described as being dead to the world. This belief that sleep is all-consuming was probably connected to the idea that sleep was a comprehensive state of being. In years past, most scientists regarded sleep as "a property of the whole organism. An animal was either awake or drowsy or asleep" (Krueger et al., 2008). Anecdotally, most behavior connected to sleep confirmed this view. But brain research has shown repeatedly that sleep does not occur in the brain or body all at once or even in the same way day after day. Instead, it may be started by neural segments in the brain and body that have been stimulated by the day's (unique) activities. The accumulation of these sleepy localized neural segments may then lead to a neural tipping point that moves an organism toward sleep (Krueger et al., 2008).

Further supporting this view that sleep is not a comprehensive state comes from correlating scientific data with other observed sleep behavior: "The often cited example of a parent arousing at a baby's whimper but sleeping through a thunderstorm dramatizes the ability of the sleeping human brain to continuously process sensory signals and trigger complete awakening to significant stimuli within a few hundred milliseconds" (Siegel, 2009). Some animals can paradoxically be even asleep and awake (as the terms are popularly understood) simultaneously. For example, dolphins and seals can be in what we might define as a state of sleep while they are simultaneously in a state of movement. Dolphins are even able to avoid objects in their sleepy path (Siegel, 2005).

Looking more broadly at the patterns of sleep in humans and other animals, some researchers have begun to see how sleep can be described as adaptive inactivity. As Jerome Siegel (2009) explains, sleep can be understood "as a state that increases the efficiency of behaviour by regulating its timing and by reducing energy use when activity is not beneficial." Seen through this evolutionarily friendly lens, sleep is one of many states of dormancy that are common in plants and animals. The spectrum of dormancy begins on one extreme with hibernation and torpor (periods of greatly reduced metabolic rates, ranging from months in bears to hours in some bats and rodents), and sleep (as experienced by dogs or humans, for example). Toward the other extreme, one can find animals that experience short periods of sleeplessness (e.g., the walrus), reduced sleep over a long period of time (certain birds during migration), or constant activity for an extended period (e.g., killer whale mothers and their calves; Siegel, 2009).

Comparing daily sleep patterns of humans and other mammals, one finds evidence of how sleep may be constructed around times that are particularly useful to a particular species. One might assume that mammals within the same order (such as primates or insects) would have consistent sleep patterns because of their similar physical and genetic characteristics. But this does not hold true. What does seem to make more sense is that sleep patterns are shaped around the particular environmental needs of any animal. Jerome Siegel points out that the big brown bat sleeps for up to 20 hours a day. This seems to correlate to the availability of its preferred meal: flying insects that are active during the few hours preceding and following daybreak. Animal sleep patterns vary widely. Siegel (2009) reports that lions "sleep long and deeply, whereas one example of their prey, giraffes, have one of the lowest recorded sleep durations and must not sleep deeply if they are to survive." For species as varied as bats and giraffes, sleep duration seems shaped by prevalent environmental conditions: limitations (for giraffes) or opportunities (for bats).

For humans, sleep can be seen as enabling sophisticated mechanisms of adaptation. On a neurological level, the neurons and neural networks in the human brain are potentially constantly changing due to learning and adapting to new environmental realities. Sleep, according to one researcher, is a process that can "stabilize, and thus preserve, functionally synaptic networks" (Krueger et al., 2008). Dreaming can be seen as another means of adapting to the environment. But instead of adjusting to past events, dreaming helps us to deal with the future in a better way. "What we may need to navigate our waking world," writes J. Allan Hobson (2009), "is an infinite set of charts from which we may draw the one best suited to an equally infinite set of real-life possibilities."

Seen in this evolutionary sense, sleep-deprived adolescents are actually being deprived of tools that could enable them to adapt to their new circumstances. This seems all the more vital at this stage of life when the brain itself is in state of tremendous upheaval and change. Couple that with the academic, social, and sexual changes they must face in the environment around them, and one can understand why adolescents have a strong need for sleep.

CAUSES OF SLEEP DIFFICULTY FOR ADOLESCENTS

Sleep disturbances in adolescents can lead to harmful effects on mood, behavior, performance, social function, physical health, and focus in class (Stores, 2009; Banks & Dinges, 2007; Curcio, Ferrara, & De Gennaro, 2006). Although sleep disorders are fairly common in adolescents, they are often underrecognized and, when they are seen, the disorders can be misleading. For instance, some children who feel sleepy during the day become more active than normal. This can lead to a misdiagnosis of ADHD (Stores, 2009).

The most common sleep disorders in adolescents include:

- Insufficient sleep
- Circadian (biological clock) rhythm disorder
- Insomnia
- Snoring
- Sleep apnea
- Narcolepsy
- Movement disorders such as restless legs syndrome
- Sleepwalking
- Bedwetting

Causes for sleep disorders in adolescents can also be behavioral. These causes include depression or anxiety, caffeine and nicotine use, or intentional sleep-phase delay to avoid school (Moturi & Avis, 2010).

Even though adolescents require between 9 and 10 hours of sleep per night, they rarely get that much sleep. Adolescents' normal sleep times shift a couple of hours later in the evening: They tend to get sleepy later (around 11:00 P.M.) than when they were young children. Left to their own devices, most adolescents would stay in bed sleeping until at least 8 or 9 o'clock in the morning. Unfortunately, schools' anachronistic starting time punishes adolescents unnecessarily, but little has been done to delay starting times to conform to adolescents' natural circadian rhythms. Actually the total sleep time of adolescents decreases to 6.5 to 8.5 hours during school nights with delayed bedtimes. As a result, daytime sleepiness and insomnia symptoms are common among adolescents (Brand et al., 2010). While it is very common in the United States for adolescents to sleep late on weekends or during holidays to make up for lost sleep during the school year, this causes more long-term problems. The contrast and irregularity in sleeping hours results in adolescents having greater difficulty in getting to sleep during the regular school week.

All these physical, neurological, and institutional challenges are compounded by another factor: parental performance. Parents may not recognize a sleep problem when it happens, or many may not seek out help when they should. And parents going through their own emotional problems can cause their children distress, which can also result in difficulties sleeping (Stores, 2009).

Overall, the statistics about adolescent sleep health in the United States are discouraging. Up to 80% of the adolescent population gets less sleep than they should, with 25% getting less than 6 hours of sleep. Many adolescents, around 25%, fall asleep in class at one time or another. Many adolescents precede their teen sleep problems with early childhood sleep issues. A survey in the early 2000s concluded that 50% of community-based pediatricians prescribed sleep medication for young children.

THE IMPORTANCE OF TWO TYPES OF SLEEP FOR ADOLESCENTS: REM AND NREM

There are two types of sleep: non–rapid eye movement (NREM) sleep and rapid eye movement (REM) sleep. NREM sleep is divided into stages 1, 2, 3, and 4. Each stage represents deeper sleep and each has unique characteristics including variations in brain wave patterns, eye movements, and muscle tone. The third stage of NREM sleep is often called deep sleep, a period when the body recovers through cell and tissue repair, including bones, blood, and immune system. As a person ages, periods of deep sleep shorten, which is why older people are lighter sleepers. REM sleep, on the other hand, is a state of dreaming. Typically, we cycle between NREM and REM sleep throughout the night, with the periods of REM lengthening as we get closer to waking up. As with the deep-sleep stage of NREM, REM sleep periods also decrease with age. For example, a baby can spend up to 50% of its sleep time in REM, compared to an adult, who spends 20% (WebMD, 2014). Despite their different characteristics, both REM and NREM sleep are linked to maintaining learning and memory (Curcio et al., 2006).

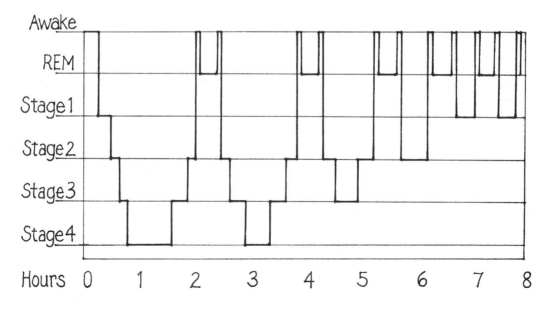

The daily rhythms of physiology and behavior (circadian rhythms) regulate the sleep-wake cycle. Irregular cycling and/or absent sleep stages are associated with sleep disorders (Institute of Medicine, 2006).

There are distinct changes from infancy to adulthood in how sleep is initiated and maintained, as well as the percentage of time spent in each stage of sleep and overall sleep efficiency. The usefulness of sleep for human development and successful aging may depend on sleep efficiency, that is, how much of sleeping time you actually spend asleep.

A dual relationship exists between puberty development and sleep during the adolescent years. Slow-wave sleep in Stage 3 and sleep latency time in Stage 4 progressively decline with advancing pubertal development; however, time spent in Stage 2 increases. These changes are thought to be due to puberty and hormone changes that happen at the onset of puberty. As an example, at mid-puberty, there is greater daytime sleepiness than in the earlier stages of puberty. Afternoon sleepiness is greater (than that in late afternoon and evening) in more mature adolescents than in younger children. With increasing age, the total time spent sleeping decreases, as does REM sleep. If bedtime is fixed, the duration of REM sleep remains constant (Colton and Altevogt, 2006).

SIGNS AND SYMPTOMS OF POOR SLEEP

The most common sleep disturbance seen in adolescents is delayed sleep phase syndrome (DSPS; Moturi & Avis, 2010). Adolescents with DSPS have great difficulty falling asleep at a determined bedtime and are unable to awaken at a desired time in the morning. Sleep problems can result in delayed bedtime, delayed sleep onset, earlier sleep offset during school days, reduced sleep duration, chronic sleep deprivation, and excessive daytime sleepiness. Many adolescents with DSPS will sleep late into the morning or early afternoon when they have the opportunity, such as weekends or holidays.

Sleep disorders in adolescents can complicate other conditions such as obesity and asthma, as well as psychological problems including depression, anxiety, and substance abuse. Affected neurobehavioral functioning is often a sign of chronic sleep deprivation in adolescents (Sadeh, 2003). This can often manifest in several function domains: memory skills, attention, motor function, and hyperactivity. Studies show that chronically disrupted sleep in adolescents can lead to problems in cognitive functioning including ability to focus, learning, and memory (Moturi & Avis, 2010). Sleep disorders can also have a negative impact on a child's mood and behavior (Mindell, Owens, & Carskadon, 1999).

TREATMENT PROTOCOLS AND SUPPORTIVE THERAPIES

The causes behind difficulty sleeping can vary widely for adolescents. The problems can originate in school with academic pressures or underdiagnosed learning disabilities. Other issues range from physical problems like sleep apnea to family issues to misuse of stimulants like caffeine. Because of the complex web of issues that can underlie sleep difficulty, it is most important that adolescents are screened for the underlying causes that can create sleep disorders. Behavioral interventions including a consistent sleep-wake schedule 7 days a week are of prime importance in this type of treatment. Use of drugs like antidepressants, while certainly appropriate in many situations, should not be the first line of defense for this complex phenomenon.

Several types of CAM treatments can have positive effects. Because of their ease of use and their gentleness, these therapies can have a calming and helpful effect on adolescents and may help them sleep better as they search for the main causes of their sleep problems. In some cases, the calming effect of these therapies may help to significantly dampen the amplitude and frequency of sleeping difficulties.

Herbal Treatments

Herbal teas are known to help us relax. Herbs such as chamomile, lemon balm, and valerian are associated with treatment of insomnia and relief of other sleep problems.

Aromatherapy

Natural oils from plants can have a calming and gently sedative effect. Lavender essential oils diffused in the air of a bedroom or on bedsheets has been effective in helping to induce sleep.

Acupuncture

Although the precise mechanisms and neuronal pathways are not known, both acupuncture and acupressure appear to have relaxing effects on the anxiety associated with insomnia (Lin 1995). Acupuncture treatments several weeks in duration can actually increase melatonin levels that are associated with the onset of sleep—this benefit is also seen in meditation, mentioned below (Spence et al., 2004). Practitioners often combine acupuncture with other treatments, such as herbs, teas, or relaxation exercises in the treatment of sleep disorders.

Relaxation and Meditation for Sleep Disorders

Quieting the mind through meditation has often been an effective treatment for insomnia. While this is not an easy thing to do right away, after several weeks of learning techniques, adolescents can often master it. Growing research evidence continues to support the value of meditation for treating sleep disorders. Regular meditation, alone or as part of a yoga practice, often results in higher blood levels of melatonin, an important regulator of sleep. Melatonin is a hormone produced in animals and plants. It is synthesized by the pineal gland in humans and plays a critical role in the regulation of the sleeping and waking cycle (Altun, 2007). Additional techniques for relaxation are aimed at relaxing muscles because increased muscle tension and intrusive thoughts interfere with sleep. Progressive muscle relaxation and biofeedback (teaching people how to better regulate their own natural functions, such as breathing or heart rate) are two alternative therapies that often provide positive results.

Exercise

Regular exercise is recommended for everyone and especially adolescents, for whom the exercise is known to deepen sleep. One study reported, "Chronic vigorous exercising is positively related to adolescents' sleep and psychological functioning" (Brand et al., 2010). This study also reported that males with low exercise levels have a risk of increased sleep disorders and less than adequate psychological functioning.

HELPING CAROLINA

As was the case with many of my patients who found success with alternative therapies, Carolina began treatments with an open mind. She was already familiar with acupuncture. She had an aunt who had gotten it in the past, so she was comfortable with it as well as with acupressure points.

She was really open to yoga positions because she was confident that she could do them at night. For instance, while lying in bed she would do a forward bend and grab her toes. Another one was Child's Pose, a sort of fetal position with the front of the forehead touching the ground. It was easy to do in bed. The key was providing techniques for her that were easy to do, so that she would be more likely to actually do them.

She also liked the idea of aromatherapy oils. She could easily spray them in the room or put them on her bed, and they would help her to go to sleep. Her favorite aromatherapy was lavender oil. I showed her some of the research studies that gave an evidentiary basis for using lavender oil for sleep. That gave her an added assurance that this had some legitimate chance of helping her. Plus, she really liked the scent.

To augment the calming effect of these treatments, I also shared some techniques of guided imagery, which aided her, in a step-by-step fashion, to slowly take her mind off the host of issues racing in her head. The next step would take her toward a calm feeling of safety and relaxation.

She would start by closing her eyes and thinking of an utterly relaxing, soothing place. For her it was a sandy beach. She had never been to the tropics, but she envisioned that location as a low-stress, soothing, and calming environment. She also liked being by the water. She would envision the waves lapping up against the shore. So she would start with that for a minute or two. This would function to get her into that safe, comfortable, calm mental space.

Then, after getting her to a peaceful environment through her imagination, we would then focus on calming her body through a "body scan." Step by step we would go from top to bottom: calming her brain and her thoughts, and relaxing her eyes. Then we would focus on different organ systems and body parts and relax those muscles all the way down. That would put her in a very calm state; it would help her to clear her mind of those other troubling thoughts because she was to focus on this activity and nothing else.

With some experience, she became very familiar and confident with the entire process. Soon, she took the initiative to design her own sleep program, integrating those holistic approaches that she found most helpful for her. She had her own little checklist that she would follow when she needed. If she woke up, she could turn to that checklist in the middle of the night to help her calm herself down again and lull herself back to sleep. By the end of the time she was in my clinic, she had overcome the most difficult step in this self-administered treatment: just practicing and making it happen so that it comes naturally. Doing it automatically reduces stress even further because you don't have to think too much about it.

After the first month, Carolina found that she was not only falling asleep faster but also waking up less frequently at night. Certainly, she would some-times have breakthrough symptoms, such as when she had a big test. But in general she was having much more restful sleep. Her mom, at one point, clearly felt that her daughter was sleeping better during the night and appeared more rested during the day.

By that time, I left Carolina to move forward with her own treatment program, although she certainly knew that she could come back whenever she wanted to. She was confident, and I was too, that she could just move on and engage in self-care techniques to ease and address her symptoms (for further discussion on how to get a teenager to commit to better sleep habits, see Chapter 3).

CHAPTER 5 SLEEP SENSORY TREATMENT PROTOCOL*

Touch: Acupressure Points**—HT7, GB41, KI3

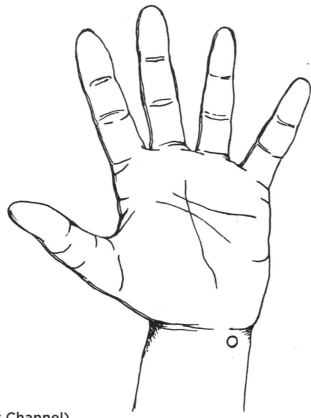

HT7 (Heart Channel)

At the major crease of the wrist on the radial side (side of wrist where the little finger is located) you can feel a tendon (flexor carpi ulnaris). Move your finger just past that tendon to the inner part of the wrist crease. You will feel a slight depression in an area of soft tissue. That is where you will find H7.

*Please refer to the Treatment Protocol Information and Resource Guide of this book (page 197) for additional detailed information on how to self-administer all sensory treatments and for added resources to locate these integrative therapies online and in local communities.

**For all acupressure points: Once you locate the point, stimulate it by pressing down with your index or middle finger and provide moderate pressure. Rotate your finger in a circular motion while pressing over the point. Continue to stimulate or massage the area for 2–3 minutes. Can be repeated as needed.

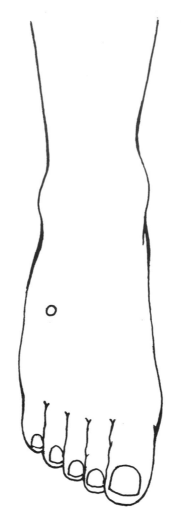

GB41 (Gallbladder Channel)

Palpate the depression distal to the base or junction of the fourth and fifth metatarsal bones, on the lateral side of the tendons (they are part of the long extensor muscles of the toes) near the little toe.

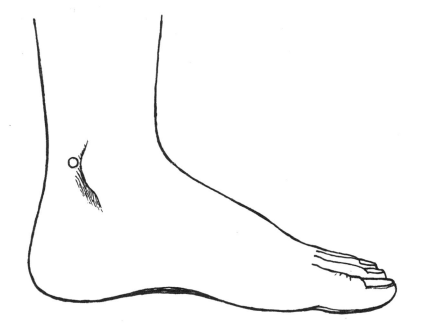

KI3 (Kidney Channel)

The midpoint connecting the greatest prominence of the medial malleolus (inner side of the ankle joint) with the Achilles tendon.

Smell: Herbs, Flowers, Plants, and Essential Oils*— Lavender and Chamomile

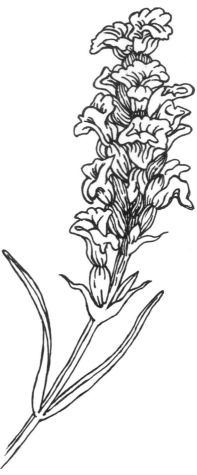

Lavender (*Lavandula officinalis*)

Lavender is one of the safest and most widely used essential oils in aromatherapy. In a 2005 study at Wesleyan University, patients sniffed lavender before sleeping. The result: increase in their amount of deep sleep, scientifically known as slow-wave sleep (Johannes, 2010).

*Essential Oils (EO) have several methods of use. Please refer to the Treatment Protocol Information and Resource Guide of this book (page 197) for additional detailed information on aromatherapy.

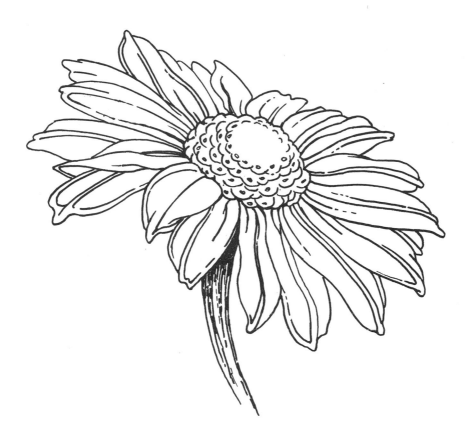

Chamomile (*Anthemis nobilis* and *Matricaria chamomilla*)

Chamomile in tea form has sedative qualities known to aid sleep and relaxation, and it also works as an essential oil delivered through aromatherapy. It smells more like apples than a flower. Its name is derived from the ancient Greek word, *Chamomaela*, which means "earth apple." Since the time of ancient Egypt chamomile has been held in high regard for its calming qualities. Chamomile flowers look like daisies, and are most commonly seen in two varieties, German Chamomile (*Matricaria chamomilla*) and Roman Chamomile (*Chamaemelum nobile*). Its dried flowers are one of the most widely used and well-documented herbs. On a cautionary note: if you have ragweed allergy, this herb may cause an allergic reaction. Although chamomile is considered a mild herb, exercise caution and check with your healthcare provider for specific health conditions. (Avallone, et al., 1996; Awad, et al., 2007)

Taste: Herbal Tisanes*—Valerian and Lemon Balm

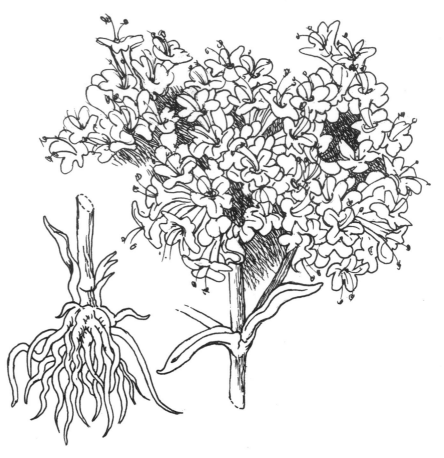

Valerian (*Valeriana officinalis*)

Valerian is known for its great calming and sleep-inducing effects as well as for a not-too-pleasant odor. (The ancient Greeks gave it the onomatopoeic moniker *phu*.) In addition to insomnia, it is helpful to counter nervousness, which contributes to sleep difficulty. It's cultivated in northern climates that are not too cold and in similar climates in the Andes. In some studies, valerian has been reported as better than placebo, but the evidence remains inconclusive. But, for those who have found it helpful, it seems that it should be used for more than 2 weeks to achieve the desired effect.

*Tea and herbal tisanes are easy to prepare and find at local stores and markets. For detailed information on preparation and sourcing please refer to the Treatment Protocol Information and Resource Guide on page 197.

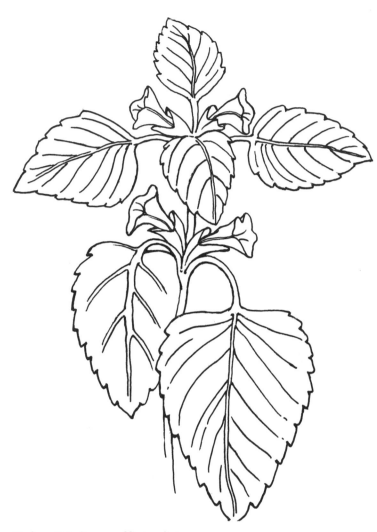

Lemon Balm (*Melissa officinalis*)

For sleep, lemon balm helps a variety of problems related to nervousness or stress, such as a racing heart or digestive problems. Lemon balm is native to the Mediterranean and it was the Arabs who first touted its health benefits centuries ago. The white flowers of this plant attract bees. Hence the genus name, *Melissa,* is derived from the Greek word for "honey bee." Lemon balm is a member of the mint family and it is associated with being a calmative. Some studies have highlighted the use of lemon balm to help those with insomnia as well as being supportive of overall sleep quality and quantity. It has been combined with valerian for added benefit. (Cases, 2010; Cerny & Shmid, 1999)

Sight: Yoga Postures—Standing Forward Bend, Child's Pose, Winding Down Twist

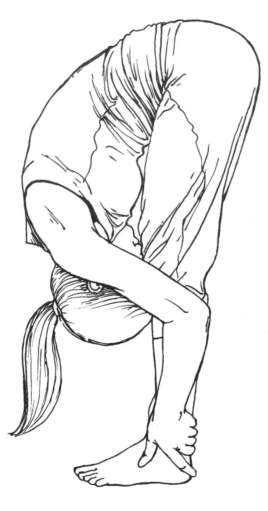

Standing Forward Bend

This is an easy pose that rewards an easy and patient approach. The forward bend is pretty straightforward. The therapeutic benefits really begin to accrue as you deepen the pose with each breath. As you inhale, you should try to lift your chest/torso a little bit and then release and get more fully into the pose with each exhalation. Besides the general relaxation this pose generates, it's great for stimulating digestion, thus helping to alleviate any digestive problems that may get in the way of sleeping.

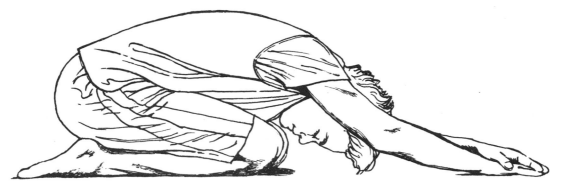

Child's Pose

Child's Pose is great for kids, especially younger kids who might feel challenged or awkward doing other yoga poses. It's a very relaxing pose and easy
to engage in. The greatest relaxation benefits, as with many poses, come with
mindful breathing. Six breaths in this pose
should be good to start welcoming sleep.

Winding Down Twist
(Also Known as Half Twist)

The majority of yoga poses
bend the spine forward or
backward. This one moves the
spine laterally in a twist. Starting in a seated position (with
legs crossed on the floor),
keep your spine erect through
the pose. Twist to one side
and then the other. Continuing
with a steady breath, deepen
the twist with each exhale.

Note on Yoga
for Sleep

Using these poses and
related poses together offers
a more complete relaxation
regimen for sleep.

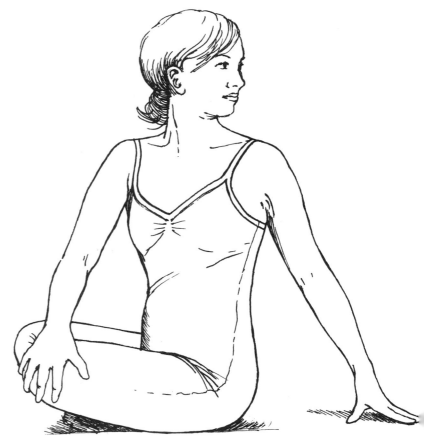

Sound: Soft Music, Soothing Melodies, Nature Sounds

An increasing number of studies have pointed to the effectiveness of music as a bridge from waking to sleep for people experiencing difficulty sleeping. Generally, a patient will want to use soft and soothing music and even gentle natural sounds like birds chirping or flowing water. In the case of music, it should be sedative, with a rhythm ranging from 60 to 80 beats a minute. The melody should be calm and regular. Usually, music to encourage sleep should be started 30 minutes before going to bed. One important additional instruction is that patients should not worry about turning the music off (Harris, 2014).

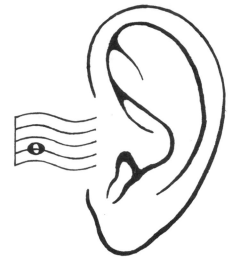

Focus and Concentration

///

JOANNA: TROUBLE ON THE SIDELINES

Joanna, who was 18 years old, had been diagnosed with attention deficit disorder (ADD) in adolescence. She had been treated for her condition, but when she came into our clinic, she had stopped her medications altogether and was looking for alternative methods. Because the principle of our practice is to complement medical treatment, our patients are never counseled to decline or cease using pharmaceuticals. Joanna had previously stopped medications under the guidance of her doctor.

Joanna was a track and field athlete, who often found it difficult to regroup and focus for practice at the end of a long school day. Although she often had difficulties focusing in academic settings as well, she was most concerned with her performance in sports. The desire to improve in sports or athleticism is not an uncommon motivator for teens seeking help. Coincidentally, many professional athletes use self-administered techniques such as meditation and massage to get centered before a game or competition.

Joanna reported that she had difficulties getting into the right mental "zone" before a track meet and was interested in learning exercises that might help her feel less scattered and more grounded.

TROUBLE CONCENTRATING: NOT JUST ADHD

Little kids often have lot of energy they need to expend in one way or another. We've all seen our own kids or those of others, for instance, running around a supermarket or restaurant, hoping to start a game of catch me if you can with a parent or older sibling. A common remark from people observing this child might be, "Oh boy, that kid is hyper!" But being hyperactive and having a lot of energy can be two entirely different things.

This semantic confusion that elides the two conditions can cause problems when people confuse normal childhood behavior with real medical conditions such as ADHD. As defined by the Mayo Clinic (2013a), ADHD is "a chronic condition that affects millions of children and often persists into adulthood. ADHD includes a combination of problems, such as difficulty sustaining attention, hyperactivity and impulsive behavior. Children with ADHD also may struggle with low self-esteem, troubled relationships and poor performance in school. Symptoms sometimes lessen with age."

Today, the *DSM-5* recognizes three types of ADHD: inattentive, hyperactive-impulsive, and combined. The designation "inattentive" is what was formerly called ADD. Some children who are diagnosed with ADHD grow out of their hyperactive traits by adulthood. Indeed, it is possible to experience inattention, distraction, and concentration problems without ever exhibiting hyperactive traits (Healthline.com, 2015). Using today's *DSM-5* criteria, Joanna would likely fall into the ADHD-inattention category.

It's important to remember that ADHD can spur many related problems (or comorbidities), such as depression. So therapists and medical professionals have to be careful to avoid both under- and overdiagnosing ADHD. Moreover, ADHD is a condition that often is not totally cured; however, one can improve the quality of life for patients by mitigating symptoms. One advantage of holistic treatments for kids having problems with focus and concentration is that these treatments can help many kids improve their ability to concentrate, whether or not they have ADHD.

Whatever degree of difficulty a child may have naturally in maintaining focus for some extended period of time, today's technologies have increased potential distractions exponentially from just 10 or 15 years ago. There are attention-grabbing activities such as checking social media sites, playing online or video games, searching the web, texting, and watching videos on YouTube. In fact, adolescents use the Internet more than any other age group today.

As Daniel Goleman (2013) explains, much Internet content falls into the category of sensory distractions. These are generally superficial and quite common. The other kinds of distractions are emotional distractions, which might be described as the thoughts going on in your head about yourself or things happening in your life. These emotional distractions are the ones that trouble people the most.

Especially troubling—and distracting—is the combination of wireless technology and the age-old problem of social anxiety among teens. Adolescents are particularly sensitive to and interested in social interactions with their peers as well as the social climate of their neighborhood and school. Both of these interests can become amplified greatly by technology. Sometimes, adolescents find these amplifications interesting and exciting and take the opportunity to text their friends with the latest gossip well into the night. Sometimes, social media platforms can be much less attractive and can cause great anxiety, such as when adolescents become victims of cyberbullying. In these and many other cases, social media can (and does) increase the scale of distracting interests and concerns for the average teen.

Another distraction that has taken hold of teens in the United States and developing countries is anxiety caused by increased competition. Globalization has not only had an impact on the labor force, but also, at least in the United States, has affected higher education. Many of the best schools now recruit students from around the world, and talented teens from the United States find it harder to get into the top schools. This pressure trickles down to the second-tier schools, thus making academic competition more stressful than ever. Other competitive situations, like sports or social popularity, can put additional stress on young people. Tiredness and emotional stress from this competitive environment can cause concentration problems in persons of any age, not just adolescents. But for adolescents, high school is probably the first time they've had to deal with the stress of competition with high stakes.

As mentioned above, ADHD is certainly not the source of or reason for all problems that are related to difficulties in maintaining focus. Other causes can include consumption of alcohol, bipolar disorder, concussions, depression, drug abuse, fatigue, hypoglycemia, hypothyroidism, sleep apnea, hunger, and medications.

PHYSIOLOGY OF ATTENTION DEFICITS

Lack of attention does come naturally to adolescents; it's the degree of that lack of focus that will make this trait a concern for medical professionals and caretakers.

The reason for this natural inattentiveness can be found mainly in the normal development of the human brain, specifically the frontal lobe. The frontal lobe of the human brain is well known for being a center of reasoning; it is centrally important in the process of helping us to think before we act. It is also the area of the brain that allows us to pay attention. For adolescents, this part of the brain is not yet fully developed. In fact, most of the brain development during adolescence occurs in the frontal lobe; so the ability for a young adolescent to be attentive is less than that of a normal adult.

It is not only brain development in adolescence that causes behavior challenges; pubertal hormones also affect the adolescent brain and behavior. Research shows that adolescence is a sensitive time for steroid-dependent brain organization. Variations in the timing of interactions between the hormones of puberty and the development of the adolescent brain can lead to individual differences in adult behavior (Sisk & Zehr, 2005).

SIGNS AND SYMPTOMS OF ATTENTION DEFICITS

The National Institute of Mental Health highlights inattention, hyperactivity, and impulsivity as the key behaviors of attention deficits. While these behaviors are perfectly normal for all children at times, they become more severe and occur more often for children with attention deficits. Children who have symptoms of attention deficit may exhibit the following behaviors:

- Being easily distracted and frequently switching from one activity to another
- Having difficulty focusing on one thing
- Losing interest in a task after a very short time
- Having difficulty focusing attention on organizing and completing a task
- Having trouble completing or turning in homework assignments
- Appearing not to be listening when spoken to
- Daydreaming and becoming easily confused

As noted by the American Academy of Adolescent Psychiatry, these difficulties in being attentive or maintaining attention can also result in a variety of problems, including:

- Acting on impulse and not thinking before acting
- Misreading or misinterpreting social cues and emotions
- Getting into accidents of all types
- Getting involved in altercations without considering potential consequences
- Engaging in risky behaviors and not considering the behavior's inappropriateness

One peculiar aspect of ADHD is that while some of the more obvious symptoms that present in childhood (especially physical hyperactivity) tend to diminish during adolescence, the condition can still remain and worsen over time. That is because while the basic problem of ADHD has not truly diminished, the pressures the adolescent may feel because of ADHD may steadily increase. As children move into adulthood, they are expected to act more independently. The adult supervision that was readily available in elementary school diminishes rapidly while these adolescents attend junior and senior high school. The problems resulting from an inability to focus and maintain attention now become more disturbing for kids because that inability suddenly becomes a major handicap in dealing with new, challenging situations: namely, more complicated schoolwork and social life.

A STUDY IN CONTRASTS: MINDFULNESS VERSUS DIFFICULTIES IN FOCUS AND CONCENTRATION

As discussed later in this chapter, yoga and meditation can be some of the most reliable means of improving adolescents' ability to concentrate. One of the goals of meditation—and often of yoga—is for an individual to become more mindful; in other words, by using meditative techniques, an adolescent may be able to perceive the world more clearly through a state of mindfulness. Mindfulness might be best described as "an unbiased receptivity of mind" (Brown, Ryan, & Creswell, 2007). This lack of bias means being open to seeing things in a fresh way, so as to avoid typecasting people or situations before seeing them as they unfold in the present. Meditation also teaches a person how to detach from inner voices and repetitive thoughts, thereby allowing the mind to be freer, calmer, and open to other ideas.

Being unable to focus on the present is paralleled by a lack of attention to one's inner feelings and ideas. The inability to "bring sufficient attention to oneself," write Brown et al. (2007), "tends to foster habitual, overlearned, or automatized reactions rather than responses that are . . . situationally appropriate." This description of the problems arising from a lack of mindfulness parallel many symptoms of ADHD. Some of the typical symptoms of childhood ADHD include leaving one's seat in situations where being seated is expected; blurting out answers before a question has been completed; difficulty taking turns; and interrupting others frequently (Goldman, Genel, Bezman, & Slanetz, 1998). All of these symptoms can be seen as automatic responses that dramatically interfere with being open and present in the moment and responding appropriately to specific situations.

Yoga and meditation can cultivate the kind of mindfulness that eases the distracted or automatic behavior of those who have trouble maintaining concentration (Brown & Gerbarg, 2012). One study looked at the positive impact of yoga on the stresses of pregnancy. Like kids entering adolescence, women in the early stages of pregnancy are encountering very new and potentially stressful circumstances in their lives. A group of women who underwent 7 weeks of mindfulness-based yoga demonstrated measurable improvements in reducing stress and anxiety as well as the ability to reduce the back pain often associated with pregnancy (Beddoe, Paul Yang, Kennedy, Weiss, & Lee, 2009).

Due to its efficacy as a treatment method, yoga is recognized by the National Center for Complementary and Alternative Medicine (NCCAM), a division of the National Institutes of Health, as a valid mind-body intervention, and is therefore increasingly utilized among clinical populations as an alternative treatment for disease.

TREATMENT PROTOCOLS AND SUPPORTIVE THERAPIES

There appear to be many opinions on the treatment of attention deficits in adolescents. While many experts believe behavior therapy alone will work best for adolescents with attention deficits, NIMH states that approximately 60% of adolescents with attention deficits are treated with medication. In many cases, a combination of medication (stimulant medications) and behavior therapy is proven best in treatment of attention deficits in adolescents. Stimulants counteract what many believe to be at least one root cause of ADHD: a dopamine deficiency in the brain. The authors conclude: "The literature on brain imaging clearly supports the presence of abnormalities in structure (smaller size) and function (hypoactivation) of critical brain regions related to dopamine [in the case of patients with ADHD]" (Swanson et al., 2007).

Nonstimulant medications such as Intuniv, Kapvay, and Strattera are also used to treat teens with attention deficits. These medications do not have the side effects of stimulant medications, which include anxiety, irritability, and insomnia. In addition, nonstimulant medications are not habit forming and are less likely to be abused.

Alternative therapies are becoming more and more common for treatment of attention deficits, including the following:

- *Yoga and or meditation.* Regular sessions and relaxation techniques can help children relax and learn discipline to help them manage symptoms of attention deficits.
- *Special diets* that eliminate foods such as sugar, wheat, milk, eggs, and artificial colorings and additives. Caffeine as a stimulant for children can be risky and is not recommended for any adolescent with attention deficits.
- *Massage therapy* is thought to be extremely effective as a relaxation technique that helps to calm anxiety. When done for about 20 minutes twice a week, massage therapy may be helpful for attention deficits on a short-term basis.

Parental involvement is very important when attention deficit is suspected. Talking openly and communicating regularly with an adolescent experiencing concentration problems are important involvements, as well as being supportive and accepting. Some of the following actions are recommended to parents who have a teen with attention deficits (ADHD in Teens, 2015):

- Provide clear, consistent expectations, directions, and limits.
- Set a daily schedule and keep distractions to a minimum.

- Support activities where the teen can have personal success (sports, hobbies).
- Build teen's self-esteem by affirming positive behavior.
- Reward positive behavior.
- Stay calm when disciplining the teen.
- Try to ensure the teen gets plenty of sleep and set firm rules for TV watching, computers, video games, and phones.

The most popular, current treatments for attention deficits focus on reducing, not curing, the symptoms.

JOANNA: GETTING BACK ON TRACK

Because Joanna was an athlete, I expected that physical interventions would resonate most with her. So her plan included acupressure combined with yoga poses, music therapy, and essential oils.

While on the field, Joanna would do forward bends while at the same time activating pressure points on her ankles. This action looked like an ordinary stretch, so the intervention was rather inconspicuous. For music, she was instructed to choose complex tunes whose effect was to focus the mind. We also gave her soundtracks at particular frequencies that are known to promote concentration. She would put earbuds in while on the bus, in the locker room, or at home in her room. For essential oils, I gave her gauze strips infused with rosemary and basil, herbs that had the effect of clearing her mind. She found that using them on the bus, on the way to a meet, was very effective.

After only a few weeks of this self-administered treatment, Joanna reported that she was better able to block out external noises, that she felt less scattered, and (most encouraging) that she felt she was learning better and internalizing more of the physical learning she needed to progress in track and field.

As an athlete, Joanna was in tune with her body, and I think this was a key reason why she felt improvement so quickly. Soon she asked to learn about more techniques. Eventually, she used the interventions before exams and applied them to other academic and social situations.

It was most gratifying for me when Joanna contacted me a year later, from college, to tell me she was still using the techniques she learned, and was regularly going to yoga classes.

CHAPTER 6 FOCUS AND CONCENTRATION SENSORY TREATMENT PROTOCOL*

Touch: Acupressure Points**—Yintang, HN1 (Bilateral), GV20, KI6

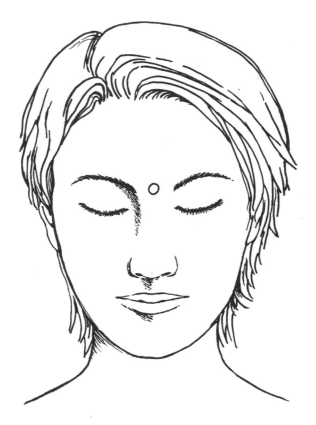

Yintang

Yintang is located at the midpoint between the two eyebrows.

*Please refer to the Treatment Protocol Information and Resource Guide of this book (page 197) for additional detailed information on how to self-administer all sensory treatments and for added resources to locate these integrative therapies online and in local communities.

**For all acupressure points: Once you locate the point, stimulate it by pressing down with your index or middle finger and provide moderate pressure. Rotate your finger in a circular motion while pressing over the point. Continue to stimulate or massage the area for 2–3 minutes. Can be repeated as needed.

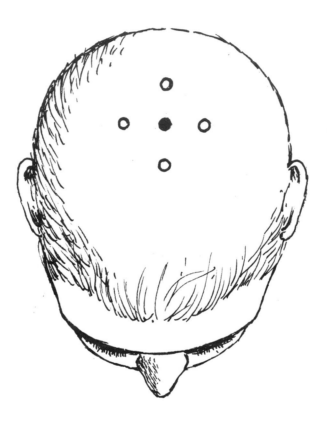

HN1 (Bilateral)

HN1 consists of four points that lie one cun (thumb width) apart from GV20 (depicted by darkened circle). One point in front, one dorsal (behind), and one point each on the lateral sides.

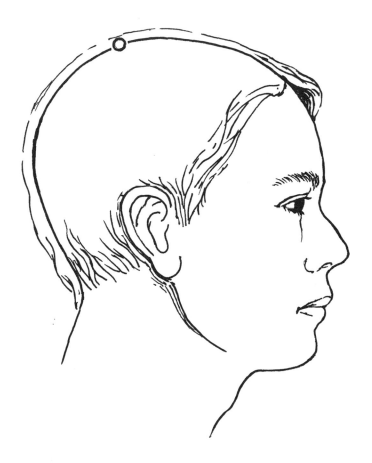

GV20

In TCM, the governing vessel (GV) or channel is thought to supply the brain and spinal regions. This point is located approximately 5 cun back along the scalp from the hairline.

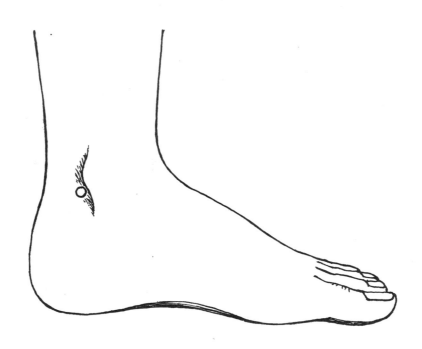

KI6 (Kidney Channel)

KI6 can be found in a depression inferior (below) the medial malleolus (inner ankle joint).

Smell: Herbs, Flowers, Plants, and Essential Oils*— Rosemary and Basil

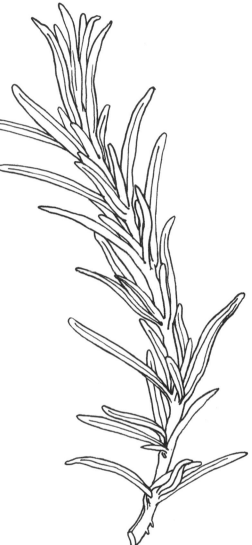

Rosemary (*Rosmarinus officinalis*)

Rosemary counteracts fatigue by helping to increase circulation of blood toward the brain, thereby improving concentration.

*Essential Oils (EO) have several methods of use. Please refer to the Treatment Protocol Information and Resource Guide of this book (page 197) for additional detailed information on aromatherapy.

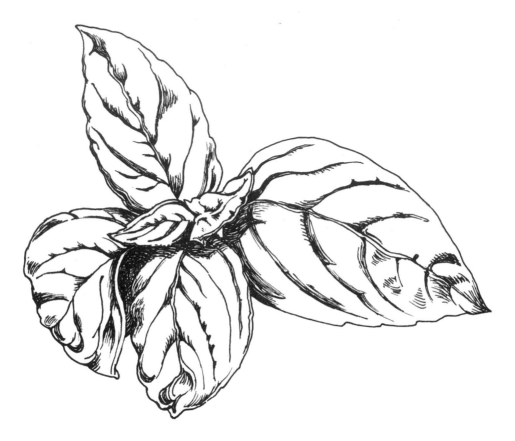

Basil (*Ocimum basilicum*)

Used in aromatherapy with other herbs like peppermint, basil has been seen to improve mental focus for people who feel acute mental fatigue. In ancient Indian (Ayurvedic) medicine, basil is considered one of the holiest and most sacred herbs. So sacred in fact, that it is often planted around temples to serve as a protector. According to modern medicine, some preliminary studies have associated basil with improving mental focus, alertness, and attention. One study combined it with other essential oils—peppermint and helichrysum—and found a beneficial effect on exhaustion. (Varney & Buckle, 2013)

Taste: Tea and Herbal Tisanes*—Green Tea and Ginger

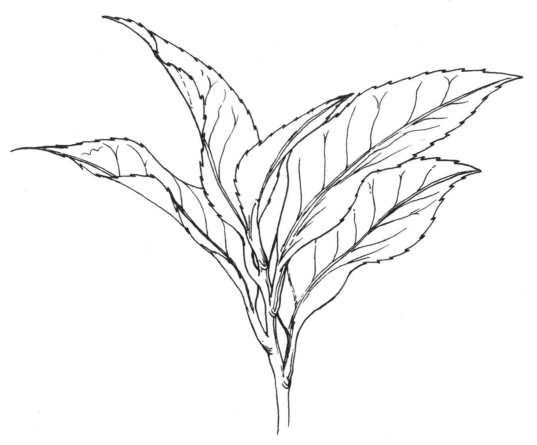

Green Tea (*Camellia sinensis*)

All true tea (white, green, oolong, black, etc.) comes from a single plant: *Camellia sinensis*. It's how the tea plant is processed that provides us with the various tea types. The use of green tea dates back thousands of years. With origins in China and Japan its application for health benefits has a long and storied history. In terms of brain health and modern science, green tea has been associated with improved focus, attention, and working memory. There are a number of healthy compounds in tea: polyphenols, theanine, theobromine to name but a few. (Schmidt et al., 2014; Kuriyama et al., 2006)

*Tea and herbal tisanes are easy to prepare and find at local stores and markets. For detailed information on preparation and sourcing please refer to the Treatment Protocol Information and Resource Guide on page 197.

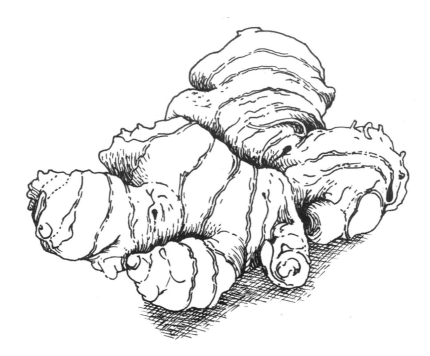

Ginger (*Zingiber officinale*)

Ginger is one of the most ancient spices used for medicinal purposes. Its wide-ranging uses are reflected in its Sanskrit name, which means "universal medicine." For teens dealing with attentional deficits, ginger may play a role in improved blood flow. Several early studies have highlighted positive effects and a supportive role in cognitive function.

Sight: Yoga Postures—Prayer Pose, Warrior 2, Eagle Pose

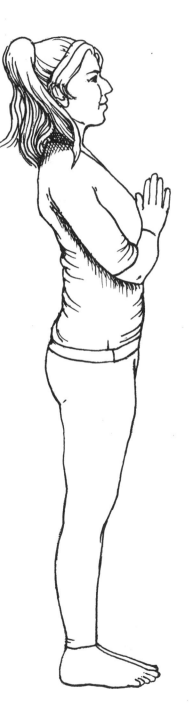

Prayer Pose

Either seated or standing, Westerners refer to this position as Prayer Pose because it resembles the common (Western) gesture of putting one's hands in front of the heart while praying. This gesture is an attempt to bring harmony to the processes that are engaged before or after a yoga session (e.g., stretching and contracting, using strength and agility). This can be seen as achieving a preparatory and necessary first step of concentration: calming the mind.

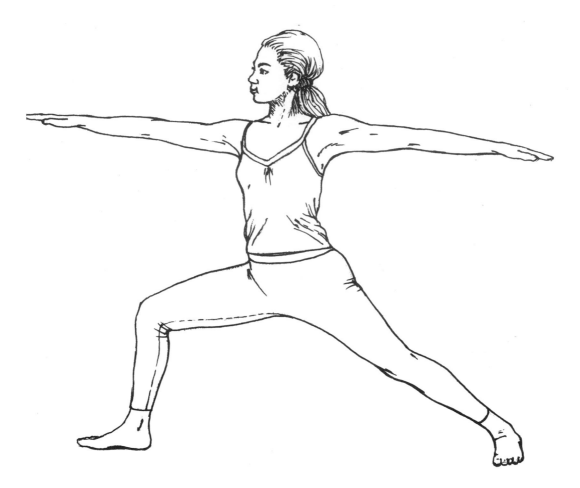

Warrior 2

Warrior 2 is a standing pose that has the primary benefit of improving concentration, because of the combination of physical strenuousness and balance it requires. The original Sanskrit name for the pose is Virabhadrasana, named after a warrior of Hindu myth, Virabhadra, who incarnated the god Shiva. You begin this pose standing with feet aligned with hips. Then, step your feet wide apart, making this one of the more dynamic yoga poses. With your heels in line, turn your front foot 90 degrees, creating a perpendicular line with your back foot. Stretch your arms wide, reaching to the horizon with your fingertips.

Eagle Pose

This kind of pose can be seen as the most challenging of the three. It's named after a Hindu myth about Garuda, the king of the birds. To do this well, one must develop balance and concentration. It engages both the upper and lower body. For the lower body, hook one of your feet behind the calf of the opposite leg. For the upper body, wrap your arms and hands together and try to have the palms touch. Hold the pose for a minute or so and then repeat on the other side.

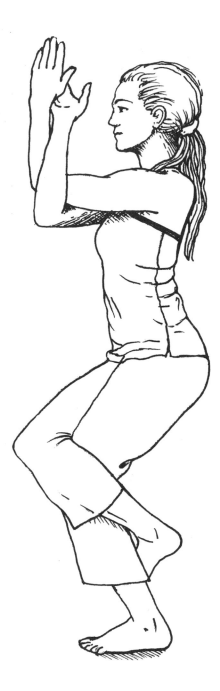

Sound: Upbeat Tempo, Major Notes and Chords, Instrumental Sounds

For those dealing with concentration problems, music has two amazing properties for therapeutic intervention. First, it engages the brain in a unique way. Neurologist and author Oliver Sacks has often been quoted as saying, "Nothing activates the brain so extensively as music." In addition to attracting the attention of the brain, music itself provides an example of order and structure, which are two antidotes to lack of attention. In the words of one music therapist, "'Music exists in time, with a clear beginning, middle, and end. . . . That structure helps an ADHD child plan, anticipate, and react'" (Rodgers, 2012). Generally, music with an upbeat tempo (at least 60 beats per minute), instrumental sounds (rather than lyrics), and a moderate noise level works best. The music should feature major notes and chords and be familiar. Avoid too many new and unusual tones. You don't want the sound to be overwhelming and complex, which becomes a distraction.

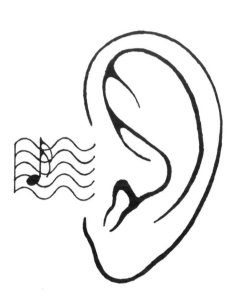

CHAPTER 7

Headache

////////////////////////

JENNIFER'S HEADACHE

It is not uncommon for some people to concentrate stress in one part of the body. One typical area is the head, and the symptom is the all-too-familiar headache. For some people, headaches are easily triggered and recurring, causing distraction, irritability, and the tendency to rely on medications to feel normal. For others, intermittent migraines can drive them to distraction, blocking out other activities for several hours or even whole days.

For 17-year-old Jennifer, a bright, sociable honor roll student, headaches were a default symptom. Various situations during the day would trigger them: classes, tests, social situations, sports practice. She could have up to five headaches in one day, or have one headache that would go on and on. Although her headaches were not technically migraines, they were chronic and required her to leave class during the day to take medications. On occasion she would have to go home in the middle of the day or not come to school at all.

She and her parents wanted other options so she would not be so reliant on NSAIDS and other pharmacological treatments over the long term. They wanted her to learn some easy management tools to help her ease her headaches.

HEADACHE: A MENTAL HEALTH AFFLICTION THAT LITERALLY HURTS

Headache is a mysterious affliction with a wide range of potential sources, symptoms, and degrees of severity. For most people who have suffered from headaches, this problem is usually temporary and not too severe. Often, headaches are caused by tension or fatigue and can be controlled by over-the-counter drugs like aspirin or ibuprofen. Sometimes they are sharp and very temporary—and almost funny. For instance, everybody has experienced that weird feeling of sphenopalatine ganglioneuralgia! Oh, sorry. Everybody has had "brain freeze," which is linked to the anterior cerebral artery of the brain experiencing a sudden increase in blood flow. This change in blood flow is caused by a sudden decrease in the temperature of the upper palate when it comes into contact with something at a very low temperature—like an ice-cold soda or ice cream—and then a surge of blood as it warms up again (Nordqvist, 2015).

These kinds of headaches, such as those caused by tension or fatigue, are called secondary headaches. As the Mayo Clinic (2013e) describes it, a secondary headache is "a symptom of a disease that can activate the pain-sensitive nerves of the head. Any number of conditions—varying greatly in severity—may cause secondary headaches." The list of conditions is, in fact, quite long. Headache can result from just about any injury or agitation of the body, from dehydration to concussions to panic attacks. In other words, outside influences that can cause a headache to start can be physical, psychological, or social. In these cases, the headache will often disappear when the primary cause is attended to: For instance, when dehydration or panic attacks end, the headaches associated with them should end too.

This is very different than primary headaches. Unlike secondary headaches, primary headaches aren't symptoms of other problems. Instead, a primary headache is caused "by problems with or over-activity of pain-sensitive structures" in the head and brain (Mayo Clinic, 2013e). Three types of the most common primary headaches are known as cluster, tension, and migraine:

Migraine: A migraine headache can cause intense throbbing or a pulsing sensation in one area of the head and is commonly accompanied by nausea, vomiting, and extreme sensitivity to light and sound. Migraine attacks can cause significant pain for hours to days and be so severe that all you can think about is finding a dark, quiet place to lie down. Some migraines are preceded or accompanied by sensory warning symptoms (aura), such as flashes of light, blind spots, or tingling in your arm or leg. (Mayo Clinic, 2013c)

Cluster: Cluster headaches occur in cyclical patterns or clusters, which gives the condition its name. Cluster headache is one of the most painful types of headache. Cluster headache commonly awakens you in the middle of the night with intense pain in or around one eye on one side of your head. Bouts of frequent attacks, known as cluster periods, may last from weeks to months, usually followed by remission periods when the headache attacks stop completely. During remission, no headaches occur for months and sometimes even years. Fortunately, cluster headache is rare and not life-threatening. (Mayo Clinic, 2013b)

Tension Headache: A tension headache is generally a diffuse, mild to moderate pain in your head that's often described as feeling like a tight band around your head. A tension headache (tension-type headache) is the most common type of headache, and yet its causes aren't well understood. Treatments for tension headaches are available. Managing a tension headache is often a balance between fostering healthy habits, finding effective nondrug treatments and using medications appropriately. (Mayo Clinic, 2013d)

The exact causes for these are not understood exactly, but studies show that people with less gray matter in certain brain structures have a higher sensitivity to pain (Zeidan et al., 2014).

The difficulty for caregivers who confront somebody with severe headache is twofold: figuring out what kind of headache you're dealing with and then figuring out the right therapy or therapies for it. Both the cause and the cure of the headache can be as idiosyncratic and unique as each individual headache sufferer. The impact of treatment can take some time to assess, so the treatment process may have many false starts. Moreover, headaches can have cascading effects, making them very hard to understand.

Let's look at these complications through the eyes of a researcher studying new daily persistent headache (NDPH), which is defined as "a daily, unremitting headache from very soon after the onset of the initial headache" (Mack, 2009). (It might also be described as the onset of chronic daily headache, or CDH, for people with no history of headache problems.) It is very common for people suffering from NDPH to have trouble sleeping, especially delayed onset of sleep. (Many other headache sufferers also share this problem.) When these kind of associated problems (or comorbidities) emerge in a patient, caregivers are presented with a tangled thread of possible diagnoses that are hard to tease out. In the case of some adolescents suffering from headaches,

> it was unclear if the poor sleep is causing chronic headaches, or if the headaches are not allowing the patients to get good sleep. It is my opinion that at the start of the CDH cycle, the poor sleep is often due to the severe headache pain. However, as the CDHs persist, usually the sleep problem becomes mutifactorial and may include pain issues, poor sleep hygiene, and a natural tendency for teens to want to be "night owls." (Mack, 2009)

But the need to find solutions, especially for children, is high. The impact of migraines, for instance, on adolescent quality of life can be tremendously costly. Severe headaches can be extremely debilitating and make a once-normal child suddenly withdraw from his usual everyday activities. Over a long period of time, this "can have significant negative psychological influences" on an adolescent's development (Kabbouche & Gilman, 2008). Indeed, in the cases of the worst kind of headache, migraine, the impact of the quality of life on children was seen to be greater than "other disease processes, including rheumatological diseases, oncological diseases, and cardiac diseases" (Kabbouche & Gilman, 2008).

Moreover, since the physical causes of severe headaches can be difficult to see, much less determine, and the onset of some headaches very sudden and dramatic (in the case of NDPH, some "patients will remember the day [and sometimes the specific hour] in which the headaches began"; Mack, 2009), families who have a child afflicted by severe headaches can be put through significant stress. They may wonder whether the child is feigning symptoms, or perhaps if the child will ever get well again.

Although conclusive proof about the origin and development of the most severe and long-lasting headaches—primary headaches—is still lacking, much of the research on the subject points to a possible combination of internal and external (endogenous and exogenous) conditions. In writing about NDPH, Kenneth Mack discusses the correlation between external factors—such as a virus or head trauma—and the onset of NDPH. Although a pattern of headaches often follows external stimuli, such as viruses, that pattern does not prove that the external influences are a "cause"; instead, Mack (2009) writes, "These factors may not 'cause' the headache, but they may aggravate an underlying predisposition to headaches. . . . [These predispositions] may be . . . a combination of host factors related to the immune system, connective tissue structure, and the familial [i.e., hereditary] nature of migraine." Some researchers believe that the origins of certain headaches can be traced to abnormal structures in the brain itself (May et al., 1999).

These findings, while not entirely conclusive, do point to a general approach to treating headaches in adults and especially adolescents, who are particularly sensitive to pharmacological interventions. This may also mean that drugs, which often are used as a temporary measure, may not be as effective for some headache sufferers in the long term. This possibility is important in light of findings suggesting that, in some cases, nonpharmaceutical interventions, such as behavioral therapies, may be at least as effective as drug therapies—perhaps even more effective.

> Although researchers have only recently begun to compare standard drug and nondrug treatments for migraine headache among pediatric populations, the available evidence suggests that the level of headache improvement with behavioral interventions may rival those obtained with widely used pharmacologic therapies. The two trials that have compared behavioral interventions and preventative drug therapies for pediatric migraine have each found behavior therapy, but not preventive drug therapy, effective in controlling migraines. (Kabbouche & Gilman, 2008)

This provides more incentive for the use of holistic treatments as a way for adolescents to cope with headache in the long term and improve their quality of life.

HEADACHES AND ADOLESCENTS

Chronic tension-type headache is the most common type of headache in adolescence; however, the International Classification of Headache Disorders noted that a majority of adolescents with CDH had headaches with features of migraine (Wang et al., 2006). Many of the risk factors for incident CDH in adolescence include female gender, acute family financial distress, obesity, higher headache frequency, and a baseline diagnosis of migraine (Lu et al., 2013). Migraine is a common problem among children and adolescents and is recognized as a significant and often debilitating condition in this population (Harding & Clark, 2014). The prevalence of migraine among young people by age 17 may be as high as 8% of males and 23% of females (Cruse, 2015).

Headache can affect all aspects of an adolescent's functioning, leading to negative affective states (anxiety, depression, anger) and increased psychosocial problems (school absences, problematic social interactions; Kabbouche & Gilman, 2008). The course of headache in adolescents is not related to age at onset, and the characteristics of the headache change over time. Hormonal factors may play a role in this (Guidetti & Galli, 2008). Migraine is considered to be a chronic disorder that can severely impact the daily activities of adolescents if not recognized and treated immediately. The impact of migraine can be measured by both the loss of ability to participate in activities and the effect on quality of life (Kabbouche & Gilman, 2008).

Physiology of Headache

Because migraine is the most common acute and recurrent headache syndrome in adolescents, it is the type of headache that attracts the most attention. Migraine in adolescents is characterized by periodic episodes of paroxysmal headache accompanied by nausea, sensitivity to light and sound, vomiting, abdominal pain, and relief with sleep. Migraine headache is usually throbbing and often unilateral. Head movement often exacerbates it. Changes in blood vessels (vascular changes) do not appear to be linked to pain, and migraine is regarded as a neurovascular headache.

Factors that influence the threshold of a person's susceptibility to a migraine attack and also the mechanisms that trigger the attack and associated symptoms may be based on anatomy and pain-producing structures within the cranium (Silberstein, Lipton, & Goadsby, 2002). Acute attacks usually occur when an individual is most vulnerable (which varies on an individual basis). It appears that the lower the threshold, the more frequent the attacks, which are triggered by internal or environmental factors that are intense enough to activate a migraine headache.

Signs and Symptoms

Young people with migraines may experience vague, uncomfortable feelings 24 hours prior to the onset of a migraine attack. This phase is called the prodrome and is not to be confused with the aura phase. The aura phase consists of focal neurological symptoms that can last up to one hour. The symptoms are referred to as "aura" because they are often visual, such blind spots or flashes of light. Other symptoms that are related to this aura phase preceding the migraine include sensory symptoms (e.g., tingling in the face) or language disturbance.

Usually within an hour of the aura symptoms improving, the typical migraine headache appears with unilateral throbbing pain and associated nausea, vomiting, and photophobia, or intolerance to light. If the migraine is not treated, the headache may last up to 72 hours before ending with deep sleep. Once the throbbing has ended, persons enter the hangover phase and may experience malaise, fatigue, and transient return of head pain in the same location for up to 24 hours. During this phase, the person may experience coughing and sudden head movement (Blau, 1992).

Adolescents with CDH often have sleep disturbance, pain at other sites, dizziness, medication-overuse headache, and a psychiatric comorbidity such as anxiety or mood disorders, and frequent school absence (Cuvellier, 2009).

Treatment Protocols and Supportive Therapies

In children and adolescents, CDH involves a multidisciplinary approach to treatment and management. Acute therapy is indicated when headache severity increases; preventive therapy is used to reduce frequency and impact of CDH; and biobehavioral therapy (which entails a patient's conscious manipulation of body processes, such as breathing) is used to assist with long-term outcome (Hershey, Kabbouche, & Powers, 2006). Additional management techniques include reassurance, explaining, education of the patient and family, and limiting medications. Pharmacological (acute and prophylactic therapies) and nonpharmacological measures (biofeedback-assisted relaxation therapy, and psychological or psychiatric intervention) are the mainstay of treatment of CDH in adolescents (Cuvellier, 2009).

Part of the education process concerning headache treatment must incorporate lifestyle adjustments, including regulation of sleep and eating habits, regular exercise, avoidance of known triggers, and stress management (Cuvellier, 2009). Progression of migraine attacks can be reversed if aggressive therapy is undertaken (Kabbouche & Gilman, 2008). Guidelines for diagnosis and treatment of headache for adolescents recommend a combination of conventional care and integrative treatment used in CAM. The recommended integrative treatments include the following (Beithon et al., 2013):

- *Acupuncture* for prophylaxis reduced the number of headaches persons had.
- *Biofeedback* can be an adjunctive therapy for migraine and tension headaches (effects were most pronounced in adolescents).
- *Cognitive-behavioral therapy* based on the premise that anxiety and distress aggravate an evolving migraine has potential for helping the person to recognize responses that may trigger a headache.
- *Physical therapy* may benefit persons through craniocervical exercises designed to correct postural faults by retraining and strengthening.

Many parents wish to avoid the chronic use of drugs with their related side effects. For these reasons, they may prefer CAM instead of a pharmacological approach. Hopefully, more physicians will be prepared to learn about CAM therapies to coordinate an integrative approach to health, especially in pediatric headache patients (Dalla Libera, Colombo, Pavan, & Comi, 2014).

HELPING JENNIFER

When patients first come into the clinic with a history of chronic or severe headaches, the first requirement is to make sure they have had a full workup to rule out any physiological or medical problems. Besides her frequent headaches,

Jennifer had a clean bill of health. Nevertheless, she did have an important characteristic: sensitivity to stimuli. She was sensitive to light, sound, and touch. Too much of any one of these stimuli would make her feel uncomfortable and could trigger headaches.

Sensory sensitivities are not uncommon among adolescents, and often a parent notices them when a child is very young. It's a hardwired trait; and when these patients understand their own sensitivities, they can then better manage their reaction to the stimuli. This information was important to know because active interventions like acupressure and yoga would not work for Jennifer. Instead, we focused on quiet, more sedentary interventions like tea or herbal tisanes, aromatherapy, and special audio tracks called binaural beats. It was important for Jennifer to do the self-help strategies in a quiet place: while lying down in bed, having a cup of tea, or staying still in a quiet place during the school day.

Jennifer started out using the techniques in the morning, at night, and whenever she felt a headache commencing. Later, she began to tune in to the happenings in her environment that were triggering her reaction and started using the interventions preventively.

Putting in a set of earbuds is a really effective and inconspicuous way for a teen to check out for 10 minutes. One interesting and effective approach uses binaural stimuli with music. Binaural music combines dissonant sounds in stereo headphones that may work to break up the electrical rhythms of a headache. It's a little bit like listening to unfinished music, but the effect can calm the mind.

Peppermint tea also had a relaxing effect on Jennifer. It was a way to stop the frenzied signals of the day long enough to calm her mind and body for a time.

To track Jennifer's progress, I asked her to keep a simple headache journal, noting the start, end, and severity of her headaches. It's important not to ask for too much documentation, because teens already have so much on their plate.

Within a few weeks, Jennifer's journal showed a decrease in the severity of her headaches but not in the frequency. By one month, the frequency started to decrease as well.

When Jennifer's sessions at the clinic ended, she felt more confident that there was another modality through which she could address her headaches. Although she still turned to medications when needed, the alternatives were at her fingertips, and she readily used them.

CHAPTER 7 HEADACHE SENSORY TREATMENT PROTOCOL*

Touch: Acupressure Points**—LI4, LIV2, GV14, ST44

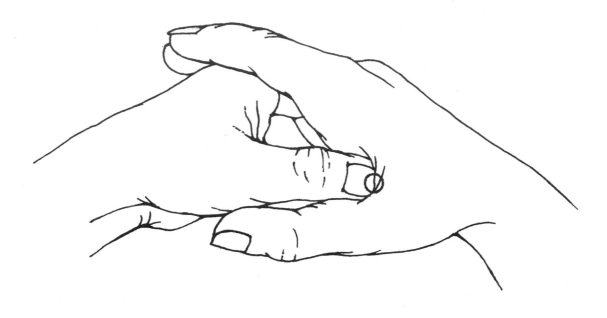

LI4 (Large Intestine Channel)

On the top side of the hand, locate the web between thumb and index finger. To find the point, squeeze the thumb against the base of the index finger. The point is located on the highest point of the bulge (fleshy prominence) of the muscle, level with the end of the crease.

---

*Please refer to the Treatment Protocol Information and Resource Guide of this book (page 197) for additional detailed information on how to self-administer all sensory treatments and for added resources to locate these integrative therapies online and in local communities.

**For all acupressure points: Once you locate the point, stimulate it by pressing down with your index or middle finger and provide moderate pressure. Rotate your finger in a circular motion while pressing over the point. Continue to stimulate or massage the area for 2–3 minutes. Can be repeated as needed.

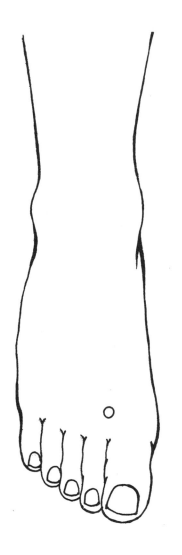

LIV2 (Liver Channel)

LIV2 is found on the foot, between the big toe and the second toe, a half thumb width from the margin of the interdigital fold or web.

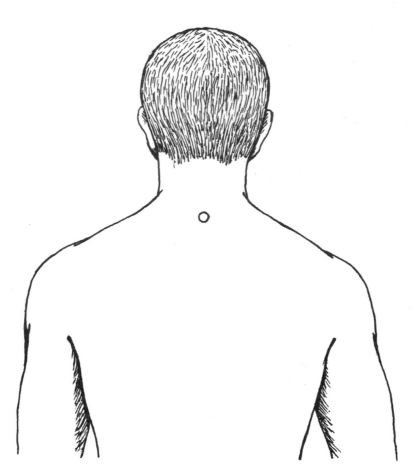

GV14 (Governing Vessel Channel)

GV14 is located inferior to the lower neck at the upper back below the spinous process of cervical spine C7.

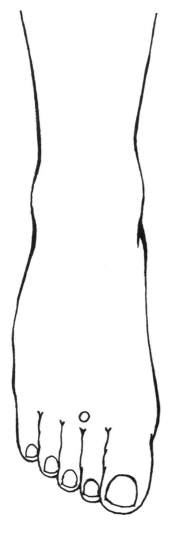

ST44 (Stomach Channel)

ST44 is found at the end of the interdigital fold (web) between the second and third toes.

Smell: Herbs, Flowers, Plants, and Essential Oils*—Frankincense and Lavender

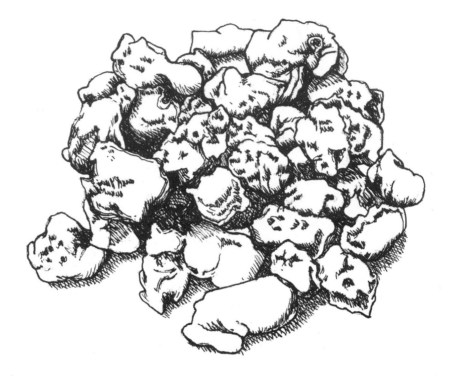

Frankincense (*Boswellia carterii*)

Made famous by the three kings who brought the baby Jesus frankincense, along with gold and myrrh, this resin is cultivated in the Arabian Peninsula and the Horn of Africa. Cultivation begins by making small cuts in the bark of the trees, which allows the sap to ooze. This sap clumps in small balls (called tears) on the bark and is cultivated regularly during the dry season in these areas, which can last 9 months. In aromatherapy, the essential oil of frankincense has been associated with sedating and anti-inflammatory properties that can relieve stress as well as headaches that come from stress.

*Essential Oils (EO) have several methods of use. Please refer to the Treatment Protocol Information and Resource Guide of this book (page 197) for additional detailed information on aromatherapy.

Lavender (*Lavandula angustifolia* **or** *Lavandula officinalis*)

A 2012 study suggests that lavender may indeed be effective in the reduction of migraine headaches (Sasannejad et al., 2010). Lavender can be delivered in several ways: as an essential oil, in raw herb form in a pouch, through an eye pillow, or in a bath.

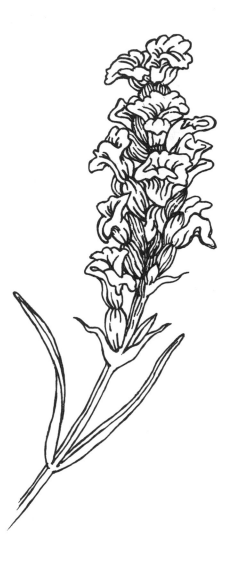

Taste: Herbal Tisanes*—Cinnamon, Peppermint, Butterbur, Feverfew Leaf

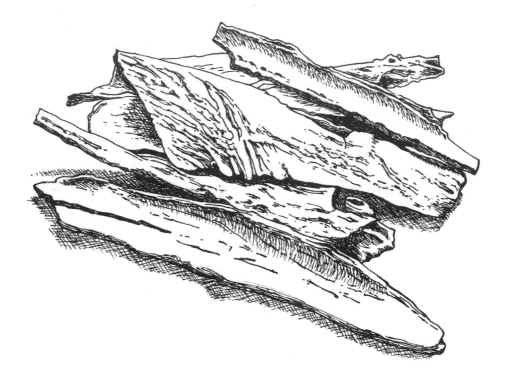

Cinnamon (*Cinnamomum verum*)

This spice is grown in the Caribbean, South America, and Southeast Asia. Long used as a culinary spice, cinnamon can be supportive to help ease an upset stomach, a symptom often coupled or associated with some headaches. It has also been touted as having anti-inflammatory properties, and the research on this spice continues to grow. (EMA, 2011; Hong et al., 2012)

*Tea and herbal tisanes are easy to prepare and find at local stores and markets. For detailed information on preparation and sourcing please refer to the Treatment Protocol Information and Resource Guide on page 197.

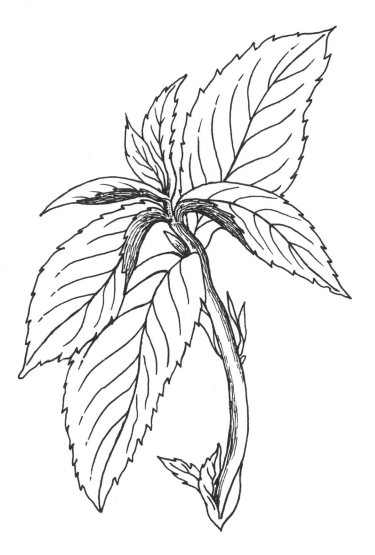

Peppermint (*Mentha* × *piperita*)

Peppermint is widely used as a healer for digestive problems. For some, stomach upset occurs along with headache. Peppermint's properties help to calm the digestive tract when it is irritated. Similarly, in several small studies, peppermint was shown to calm or ease the discomfort related to tension headaches. It's most often used as a tea.

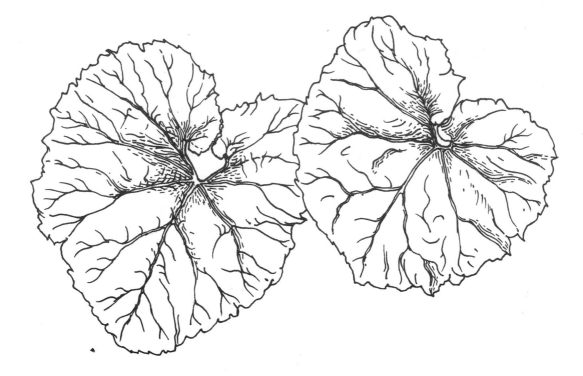

Butterbur (*Petasites hybridus*)

Butterbur grows in marshy areas in Europe, Asia, and North America. Use preparations free of the pyrrolizidine alkaloids (PAs) as they have been associated with cases of liver damage. PA-free versions are readily available and have been studied and found to be safe in children and adolescents (Agosti, Duke, Chrubasik, & Chrubasik, 2006; Pothmann & Danesch, 2005; Oelkers-Ax et al., 2008).

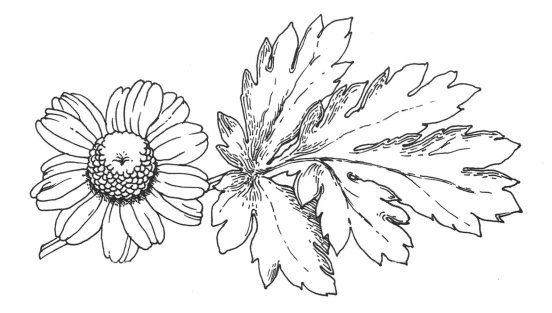

Feverfew Leaf (*Tanacetum parthenium*)

This plant is a member of the daisy family and native to southeastern Europe. Now, it is grown throughout Europe, Australia, and North America. It has been used for centuries to help ease headache and pain. There is evidence of its use in ancient Greece to reduce inflammation (Pfaffenrath, Diener, Fischer, Friede, & Henneicke-von Zepelin, 2002; Diener, Pfaffenrath, Schnitker, Friede, & Henneicke-von Zepelin, 2005).

Sight: Yoga Postures—Cat Pose, Legs Up Wall, Seated Side Opener

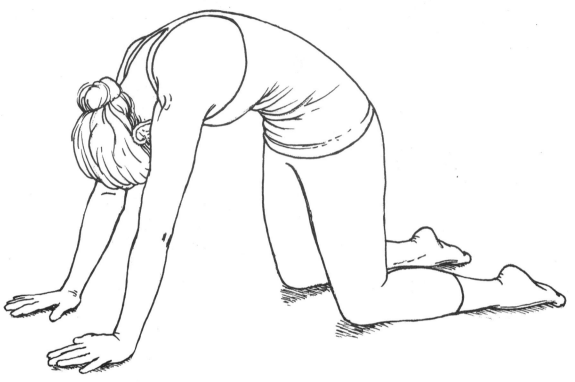

Cat Pose

Like Downward-Facing Dog, Cat Pose, does look a lot like its namesake. Now, instead of being a playful puppy, you should think of yourself as a cat stretching after waking up. The pose starts on all fours, knees below hips and wrists below shoulders; both the legs and arms should be perpendicular to the floor. Starting from this position, inhale and curve your spine upward while your head should move downward. Breathe out and then come back to the original position. This can help with headache because of the way the pose can relieve tension in the neck, shoulders, and spine.

Legs Up Wall

The passiveness of Legs Up Wall Pose is one of the reasons why it can help with headache. Not too much effort or straining involved—just lie back and enjoy the benefits, which include reducing fatigue and calming the mind.

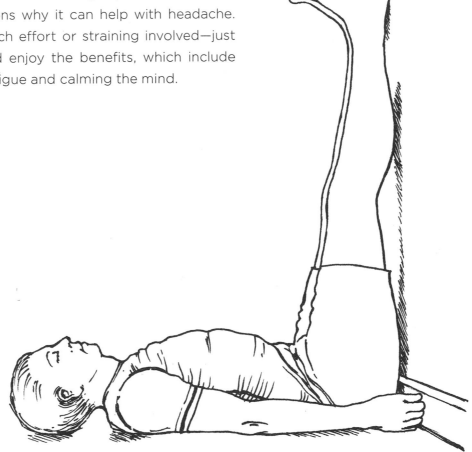

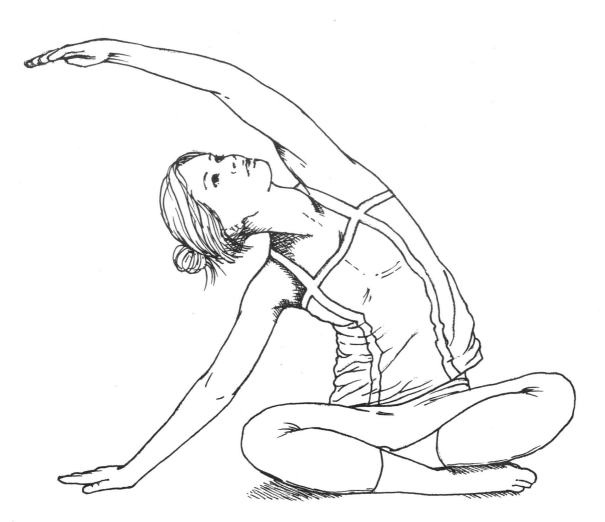

Seated Side Opener

Like Cat Pose, Seated Side Opener eases tension that can cause a head-ache—around the neck, the shoulders, and the spine. It also increases blood flow to your head. Begin this pose in a seated position, legs crossed and arms relaxed. Now, get ready to sway gently back and forth. Start with your right arm and reach upward. Take your left hand to the ground and slowly move it along the ground—all while keeping your seated position. This tension between being seated perpendicularly while moving your torso horizontally creates the opening in the side. Breathe slowly for 8 to 10 breaths, then move back to your seated position. Start the pose on the other side with the left hand reaching upward, and so on.

Sound: Calming, Uplifting Music, Self-selected Playlists

Because headaches can often be such a physical and visceral experience, it is not surprising that music therapy can be combined with some sort of physical activity in these cases. One can combine relaxation exercises, like yoga, with background music. Again, pick something uplifting or calming while doing it. In more extreme cases, like migraine, some therapists have used music in a wide variety of interventions over a long period of time, combining music with guided imagery, guided movement, tactile stimulation, daydream improvisation, body percussion, and varying the types of music (Relaxation techniques for migraines and headaches, 2015; Oelkers-Ax et al., 2008).

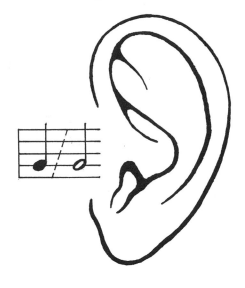

CHAPTER 8

Substance Abuse

//

JOSÉ'S TURN TO ALCOHOL

Seventeen-year-old José was in rehab for alcoholism. When he came to the clinic, he had been sober for one month and was attending a regular outpatient program. José had found the relaxing effects of beer and hard liquor too compelling to moderate; he had grown dependent on drinking before bed as well as first thing in the morning. At the peak of his addiction, he would have up to 10 beers a day and, as a result, became unable to function.

His father (who was, unfortunately, not a consistent presence in his life) also struggled with alcoholism. Thankfully, his mother was very tuned in to what was happening to her son and not only put him into rehab but came to our clinic seeking interventions that would support his recovery.

Alcohol use by minors often follows a similar pattern: usually an older sibling or a friend buys for the younger drinkers. So drinking starts out as a social activity, but, as in José's case, it may then evolve into a solitary activity. José drank to block out his feelings of powerlessness. No one in his family had ever gone to college before, and he was under internal and external pressure to be the first to succeed. He drank to fall asleep at night and to ease his anxiety about his future.

Even though he had stopped drinking, he was experiencing serious side effects, such as cravings and sleeplessness. His mother brought him to the clinic to find ways to help him cope as he tried to extinguish his habit for good.

IT CAN TAKE A VILLAGE TO SOLVE A SUBSTANCE ABUSE PROBLEM

The placement of the topic of substance abuse at the end of this book is appropriate. Why? Because substance abuse can be seen as a self-treatment of last resort. One researcher has noted that " 'problem drug use' appears most prevalent during a developmental period of 'emerging adulthood,' which approximately extends from 16 to 25 years of age" (Arnett, 2000, quoted in Sussman, Skara, & Ames, 2008). This corroborates the observation that drugs are generally a last resort for kids: younger teens or preteens dealing with headaches or stress, for instance, probably turn to drugs less than do older adolescents because either they are not independent enough to seek drugs on their own or because they may turn to familial or community supports first.

Adolescents who feel like they can't remedy their mental health problems may eventually turn to drugs and other potentially dangerous substances to find some relief from the distress they are feeling. Moreover, many adolescents experimenting with controlled substances—from the dextromethorphan in cough medicines to cocaine—often begin experimenting with small doses that can then grow into really significant, dangerous, and long-lasting usage. The high rates of relapse for supposedly cured drug users of any age also points to the need for a comprehensive plan for effective self-care that can be accessed beyond the borders of the health clinic. Some clinicians call this approach "a continuum of care" (Sussman et al., 2008). Teens can also start getting hooked on drugs through recreational use. In either case, regular abuse of drugs can lead to major physical and mental health problems.

For teens who are struggling to avoid drugs, late adolescence and early adulthood throw many new and significant challenges their way that can push them back into some sort of substance abuse. Challenges include achieving graduation, looking for a job, living with roommates, forming significant romantic relationships, and becoming financially independent, among other tests of adulthood. These multifaceted demands require that a true "holistic [recovery] process affecting many life domains" become part of the process of growth.

What this holistic approach implies is some sort of community or broad-based involvement in the recovery and maintenance of teens that have a history of substance abuse. In other words, it's hard for an adolescent to get over substance abuse without support from several networks in his or her life (Breslin, Reed, & Malone, 2003).

As witnessed in our multi-site program, the presence of school clinics that offer easy-to-administer supports for mental health problems had some surprising effects and a positive impact on the lives of adolescents. Offering a therapeutic program that caused minimal disruption to daily life created a new and welcoming community for mental health programs. For adolescents trying to cope with mental health problems, the ground beneath their feet changed in very good ways. Instead of encountering resistance or ridicule from the community, the gentle means of integrative techniques combined with its successes made family and friends first curious and then receptive to these therapies. Now, instead of potential isolation and estrangement, kids undergoing our therapies encountered curiosity and support. In some cases, they even became role models to others who needed help. Normalizing the process of recovery from mental health issues, helps adolescents and young adults see that everyone struggles with these issues on some level. When teenagers feel less alone in the experience, they will be more likely to see support from other parts of their lives, such as school, friends, church, family, clubs, teams, and the like.

Holistic therapies represent a bridge between estrangement and acceptance for adolescents dealing with substance abuse. By tending to the symptoms of substance abuse while simultaneously normalizing therapeutic interventions, holistic therapies can be effective in the long term by making it easier for adolescents to turn to community resources for help.

This represents a complete inversion of the old patterns of common community reactions to people undergoing mental health treatment: negative stereotyping and possible estrangement. Indeed, the obvious side effects of drug use and periods of inpatient care can at times create a real separation—physically and mentally—between the patient and the community. One can argue that substance abuse problems can result in longer periods of estrangement from the community or peer group than other mental health problems.

SUBSTANCE ABUSE: DANGERS AND TRENDS

Some adolescents abuse illegal drugs or misuse prescription medications or household substances once or occasionally. By twelfth grade, almost half of all adolescents have abused an illegal drug at least once. The drug most commonly used by adolescents is marijuana; however, other substances can easily be obtained by teens. Prescription medications, glues, and aerosols are always in the home (Johnston et al., 2008). But for some adolescents, drug use can take a much worse turn: problems at school and home, developmental setbacks, and, as one study noted, "Substance use and dependence are among the most prevalent causes of adolescent morbidity and mortality [illness and death] in the United States" (Sussman et al., 2008).

The substance abused most frequently by adolescents is alcohol: up to 39% of adolescents reported drinking some alcohol. Alcohol consumption is followed by 23% using marijuana, and then 16% smoking cigarettes (Johnston et al., 2008). Alcohol is perhaps the most immediately dangerous drug or controlled substance for teens because of its contribution to motor vehicle accidents involving teens, which is the leading cause of death in this age group (Hoyert & Xu, 2012). Fortunately, cigarette smoking among adolescents has declined greatly over the last 15 years; however, the use of smokeless tobacco has increased (Johnston et al., 2008). In general, the lethal outcomes connected to tobacco use mean we should not be complacent about its use among our youth. It turns out that tobacco use harms almost every organ in the human body (Brody, Beach, Philibert, Chen, & Murry, 2009). And more than 6 million children born between 1983 and 2000 will die in adulthood of smoking-related illnesses (Hahn, Rayens, Chaloupka, Okoli, & Yang, 2002).

One trend that seems to be gaining popularity is the abuse of prescription and over-the-counter drugs by adolescents, which sometimes is referred to as "pharming" (Levine, 2007). Cough medicines account for about half of the over-the-counter prescription drugs abused by teens. When cough medicines began to be manufactured in the form of gel tabs in the 1990s—thus making the ingestion of the drug easier—recreational use began to grow. The nicknames or street names of these prescription drugs (e.g., including skittles and red hots) pointed to the rapid and wide adoption of this kind of drug use among adolescents.

While cough medicines (as well as other over-the-counter drugs) are very familiar and can seem innocuous, abuse of these household items can lead to severe health consequences. Looking closer at cough medicines, one finds that a common active ingredient is dextromethorphan. While therapeutic amounts of the drug are 10–30 mg per dose, teens abusing this drug might take 100–600 mg of dextromethorphan at a time. At lower doses one might feel a mild stimulant effect. At 300 mg, a person starts to become intoxicated and experiences some hallucinations, slurred speech, and memory problems. Getting up to 600 mg, users can feel their senses off-track or altered, their eyes moving involuntarily (known as nystagmus), and sometimes feel like they are going through out-of-body experiences (Levine, 2007).

These trends in abusing over-the-counter drugs are paralleled by the general increase in prescription drugs that can be found around the house by teens, especially drugs like Adderall, Concerta, and Ritalin, which are stimulants used to treat ADHD. The general increase in the diagnosis of ADHD has led to the parallel increase in abuse of drugs like Ritalin by teens at home. On top of the euphoria Ritalin can produce, dependence can eventually occur along with withdrawal symptoms when an adolescent tries to kick the habit. All kinds of drugs easily obtained at home provide more gateways to the use of other kinds of substances whose impact on health and addictive potential grow over time.

The misuse of substances can result in a wide range of physical, social, and emotional problems, including these:

- Immediate consequences such as overdoses and accidents
- Economic problems related to purchasing substances or losing employment because of addiction problems
- Temporary physical impairment as well as permanent physical injuries or disabilities from persistent use
- Social problems, such as estrangement from family or peers or poorly developed social skills
- Legal problems, including incarceration and a permanent criminal record
- Closely related problems, such as poor academic performance, teen pregnancy, and transmission of sexually transmitted diseases
- Crimes such as stealing, vandalism, and violence associated with heavy drug use
- Disorganized thinking and unusual beliefs that may interfere with problem-

solving abilities and emotional function, leading to social isolation (Sussman et al., 2008)

The importance of arresting the rate of drug use by teens cannot be overstated. As we have seen in many of the case studies in this book, the lives of teenagers are beset with many new challenges that come at the same time these children are undergoing massive changes to their bodies and, most significantly, their brains. A perfectly healthy teen will encounter many problems and situations that will challenge her abilities and faculties as she is undergoing development. Abuse problems compound the difficulty in confronting short-term problems, which may cascade into long-term issues. Moreover, these substances have a lasting impact on the bodies and minds of teens, as well as the social skills that they will need to get along with others for the rest of their lives.

PHYSIOLOGY OF ADDICTION

Research has shown that substance abuse by adolescents may follow specific progressive patterns. Early heavy caffeine use may be a gateway drug that leads to alcohol and tobacco use, followed by marijuana. These are the first drugs of abuse that adolescents experiment with. Further data suggest that use of both alcohol and tobacco is most likely to be associated with additional substance use, such as cocaine, hallucinogens, inhalants, and black-market prescription medications (Sussman et al., 2008). As we all know, many drugs have some sort of addictive potential. In understanding the physiology of addiction, we might look at two sides of the condition: initial motivators of use and impacts over time.

Initial Motivators of Use

For a teen attracted to drug use, some of the initial motivations involve looking for something that can help to compensate for a problem or deficiency in the teen's life. Using scientific language, we might say that teens are seeking some "individual mechanism of effect" that will help to change their mood, outlook, or feelings about a situation. Teens dealing with lots of stress or tension may search for a depressant that will result in relaxation and pain relief. Examples include alcohol, benzodiazepines, and narcotics such as morphine and methadone (Miller & Giannini, 1990). Kids who feel depressed or lack energy may search out a stimulant, including amphetamines, nicotine, and cocaine, all of which stimulate the release of the reward system and cause heightened alertness and energy resulting in euphoria (a high). Once the high wears off, the user often feels depressed and wants more of the drug, thus worsening the addiction (Miller & Giannini, 1990).

Recreational drug use causes the release and prolonged action of dopamine and serotonin within the reward circuit, a network of different parts of the brain working together to reinforce behavior. Different types of drugs produce these effects through various methods; however, dopamine has the greatest effect because it binds to the D1 receptor class, which triggers a signal cascade within the cell. This cascade targets neurotransmission of what is called the direct pathway. This pathway facilitates addiction and impulsivity by positively stimulating reward areas of the brain.

The reward circuitry includes interactions between many areas of the brain, thus making it very influential in the overall functioning of the brain. One element of the reward circuitry is the prefrontal cortex, which is responsible for integration of information that is crucial in the triggering or encouragement of a particular behavior. Because the prefrontal cortex acts as the source of origination for motivation as well as a filter for stimuli to the brain (grading the stimuli on a scale, so to speak, from important to unimportant), it plays a big role in shaping behavior. Another part of the reward circuitry is the hippocampus, which is important for learning and memory. So, if the prefrontal cortex is influenced by a drug to choose a particular behavior over another behavior, and the hippocampus learns how to repeat this and remembers how enjoyable the experience was, you've got a potential addiction on your hands.

Impacts Over Time

Addiction can be understood as a downward spiral in which the body and brain attempt to compensate for stressors on the body due to the use of a drug. Those stressors are an unhealthy new equilibrium in the body that is created by consuming a controlled substance or other drug. Unfortunately, when addicts repeatedly try to get back to the new equilibrium (the high feeling) after the effects of a drug wear off, they cause an incredible amount of pain and damage to the body. In other words, the body is undergoing the feeling of an almost constant state of change. This negatively effects the body's ability to maintain a healthy equilibrium (homeostasis) and forms a new set point that can only be maintained by continued and increasing use of the addictive substance (allostasis).

During drug use, many stress mechanisms are activated. The activation of sections of the brain associated with drug addiction influences the emotional state of a drug user. As drug use escalates, so does the presence of corticotrophin-releasing factor in human cerebrospinal fluid regulating expression of stress hormones (Koob & Kreek, 2007). Increased release of stress hormones, such as cortisol, causes our body's fight-or-flight response mechanisms to be activated. In the short term, our physiology can compensate. But, when this chronic stress state persists, the same hormones that are helpful for mild or short-term stress reactions become harmful when left unchecked. Over time, chronic stress (substance abuse is a physiological stressor) contributes to an array of medical conditions that include heart disease, diabetes, metabolic dysfunctions, insomnia, and depression, to name but a few.

Drug addiction is also characterized by strong drug-seeking behaviors when the addict persistently craves and seeks out drugs, despite knowledge of harmful consequences (Kalivas & Volkow, 2005; Koob & Kreek, 2007). They are craved often because these drugs produce a reward that is euphoric. Euphoria-induced behavior is often associated with repeated drug exposure (Kalivas & Volkow, 2005; Koob & Kreek, 2007).

Addiction can damage the brain and body, especially as the reward from the drug decreases and the adolescent's ability to overcome the depressed state following drug use fades. The result is depression, which causes the drug user to take the drug again before the brain and body come down to natural equilibriums. Thus, a constant state of stress evolves and the presence of environmental stressors (such as difficulties at school) may induce stronger drug-seeking behavior (Koob & Kreek, 2007). Withdrawal happens when a person tries to adjust from the unhealthy equilibrium brought on by addiction to the natural healthy equilibrium of sobriety.

There is often an increase in sensitivity to a drug after prolonged use, which is called sensitization. A transcription factor (a protein that binds to specific DNA sequences) called delta FosB increases the user's sensitivity to the effects of a substance and can remain activated for weeks after the effects of the drug have faded. This hypersensitivity is thought to be responsible for the intense cravings associated with drug addiction, along with peripheral cues of drug use such as related behaviors or the sight of drug paraphernalia (Koob & Kreek, 2007).

A person addicted to heroin, for example, only feels whole or normal when taking heroin. But there's a dark hitch: In taking heroin to attain the new normal, many other harmful things affect the body. Heroin can change the brain itself, causing serious imbalances in hormonal and neuronal systems. There are also actual reductions of the brain's white matter. After taking heroin for a while, there is a high rate of tolerance among users, meaning that it takes increasing amounts of the drug to achieve a high over time. As the National Institute of Drug Abuse (2014) reports in a particularly sad passage, "Once a person becomes addicted to heroin, seeking and using the drug becomes their primary purpose in life."

Signs and Symptoms

Parents should be aware of some of the most common symptoms of adolescent drug abuse. There are many behavioral changes that parents may notice in their interactions with their children, including making excuses, staying in their room, breaking curfew, lying, stealing, and becoming verbally or physically abusive toward others. Parents might also observe their children experiencing mood swings and sleepless nights, and having new friends. Finally, behavioral symptoms might include physical symptoms of drug intoxication and withdrawal. There are many physical traces of drug use, especially items connected to drugs (paraphernalia such as matches, rolling papers and pipes, mirrors for drugs that are snorted, needles, syringes, tourniquets), and the smell of drugs on a person or in a room (often a marijuana odor).

Parents should know that the signs and symptoms of drug use vary greatly, depending on the type of drug being used. What are some of these symptoms and warning signs of specific drug abuse? Here are some of them:

- *Tobacco:* tobacco smell, irritability, discolored fingertips, lips, or teeth, cigarette butts at curbside
- *Marijuana:* reddened whites of eyes, sleepiness, excessive hunger, lack of motivation, excessive happiness, paranoia

- *Cold medications:* sleepiness, rapid or slowed heart rate
- *Inhalants:* runny nose, smell of gasoline or other solvent, confusion or irritability
- *Depressants:* sleepiness, lowered inhibitions, poor coordination, slowed heart rate or low blood pressure, dizziness
- *Stimulants:* rapid heart rate or high blood pressure, irritability, excessive happiness, less need for sleep, paranoia, seizures
- *Narcotics:* feeling less pain, excessive happiness, sleepiness, slowed or stopped breathing
- *Hallucinogens:* trouble sleeping, blurred perceptions, paranoia
- *Dissociative anesthetics:* higher blood pressure and heart rate, memory loss, nausea and vomiting, irritability, aggressiveness (e.g., ketamine, also known as Special K)
- *Club drugs (ecstasy):* feverish teen that does not sweat, finding multiple lollipops or other hard candies (used to guard against teeth grinding and sore jaw), the teen seeming to love everyone and/or have an excessively happy mood (euphoria)
- *Anabolic steroids:* increased irritability or aggressiveness, rapid increase in muscle definition, thinning or loss of head hair, marked increase in acne over a short period of time, finding needles (Dryden-Edwards, 2015)

Note that the physical symptoms of withdrawal from these drugs are often almost the opposite of the effects of intoxication.

Treatment Protocols and Supportive Therapies

Many treatment facilities and therapists offer an array of integrative therapies that are often used in conjunction with traditional treatments. Traditional modalities of treatment for substance abuse in adolescents may include individual, group, and family therapy; however, a holistic approach to treatment also offers patients an opportunity to develop a stronger sense of identity, self-esteem, and self-confidence. CAM therapies include a wide variety of techniques and programs: dance and movement therapy, tai chi, art therapy, leisure and recreational skills, spiritual growth and development, vocational and skill-building services, physical health and exercise programs, acupuncture, yoga, and meditation (Breslin et al., 2003).

Mindfulness meditation is a good way to regulate mood and can lower levels of the stress hormone cortisol, boost the immune system, and assist the body in detoxifying itself of harmful chemicals, which can affect neurotransmitter receptors and alter mood. An increasing number of studies indicate that mindfulness-based relapse prevention techniques do reduce cravings and prevent relapse as well as traditional treatment (Witkiewitz & Marlatt, 2005). The journal *Substance Use and Misuse* published an entire special issue in April 2014, focused on mindfulness-based interventions for substance use disorders. Mindfulness practices may also support long-term outcomes by strengthening adolescents' ability to cope with the discomfort associated with desire (Bowen et al., 2014).

HELPING JOSÉ

The alternative treatments we offer at the clinic are not a substitute for a comprehensive medical rehabilitation program. Instead, CAM therapies are employed after abstinence, when the patient is coping and struggling to stay clean and extinguish bad habits.

When treating a client with a substance abuse issue, my first requirement is that he or she must be drug free for at least one month. That was the case for José. Our focus was to directly address the side effects he was experiencing through his recovery.

It's easy to think of substance abuse being in a totally separate category from the other disorders that we see in teenagers, described elsewhere in this book. But abusing drugs is not the problem itself; it's the feelings of inadequacy, anxiety, stress, or pain that drives teens to self-medicate with drugs. Therefore, patients with drug abuse problems can often be successfully helped in a program that teaches them how to take care of the mind and body in general.

As I mentioned, the first step in wellness is for a substance abuser to stop using. When he stopped drinking, José immediately had problems falling asleep and would wake throughout the night. His REM sleep was seriously disrupted. So I introduced a nighttime routine of yoga before bed. The poses that he found most relaxing were cross-legged twists, lying on his back with legs extended against a wall, and forward bends touching toes while sitting on the floor. Other poses included Happy Baby and the morbidly named Corpse Pose. These poses were chosen because they are thought to invoke a restful state. José seemed to like doing yoga before bed and it soon became part of his evening routine.

To help address his cravings for alcohol, I recommended several teas, acupuncture, and acupressure. Teas with ginseng, thyme, or dandelion are associated with a reduction in addiction cravings. José would carry tea bags so that he could make a cup whenever he felt a craving sensation. Sometimes his use was limited by a lack of boiling water, so most often he drank tea at home in the mornings and at night.

During the 8-week program, I administered acupuncture to José on his weekly visits. Then I taught him the acupressure points that he could apply himself. In either situation—administered by me or self-administered by a patient—the acupoints remain the same. Locations on several points along the head and body help to curb cravings and can be accessed somewhat inconspicuously and, therefore, applied as needed.

By the second week of treatment it was clear that José was really taking to the new methods. As with all my patients, I want to make sure that their practice is enjoyable to them. This is important because I cannot expect compliance if there is no perceived benefit. José took ownership of his routines and, I think, genuinely enjoyed them. He started reporting less anxiety and some improvements in sleep about halfway through his treatment at the clinic. For a person experiencing regular cravings, it was helpful to have a go-to activity whenever the feelings arose. Acupressure often served as an outlet for him throughout the day. Around week 6, José felt as if he could finally get through the day feeling less miserable, and he began to focus again on his graduation goals. As we had hoped, the interventions seemed to help ease his symptoms and allow him to build long-term resiliency.

A year after he left the clinic, I learned that José graduated on schedule and soon enrolled full time at a local community college. It was a satisfying outcome for both practitioner and patient.

CHAPTER 8 SUBSTANCE ABUSE SENSORY TREATMENT PROTOCOL*

Touch: Acupressure Points**—Shen Men, Craving Point, LIV2, LU9, HT7

Shen Men

Shen Men can be found in the external upper ear in a valley called the triangular fossa. To locate this point in the outer ear, follow the antihelix (curved prominence of cartilage along the upper outer ear) upward to where it splits into an upper and lower branch. At the center of where it splits Shen Men is slightly inward and upward.

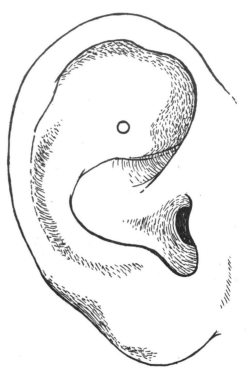

*Please refer to the Treatment Protocol Information and Resource Guide of this book (page 197) for additional detailed information on how to self-administer all sensory treatments and for added resources to locate these integrative therapies online and in local communities.

**For all acupressure points: Once you locate the point, stimulate it by pressing down with your index or middle finger and provide moderate pressure. Rotate your finger in a circular motion while pressing over the point. Continue to stimulate or massage the area for 2–3 minutes. Can be repeated as needed.

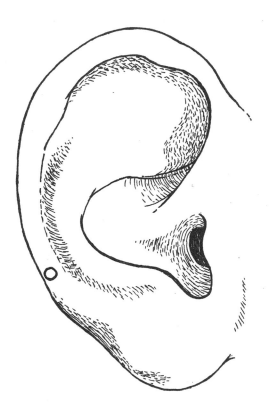

Craving Point

At the end of the postantitragal fossa at the intersection with the edge of the ear is the craving point. Start at the earlobe and move upward approximately one-third of the way along the outer cartilaginous rim of the ear.

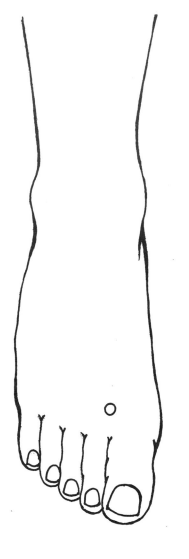

LIV2 (Liver Channel)

LIV2 is on the foot, between the big toe and the second toe, a half thumb width from the margin of the interdigital fold or web.

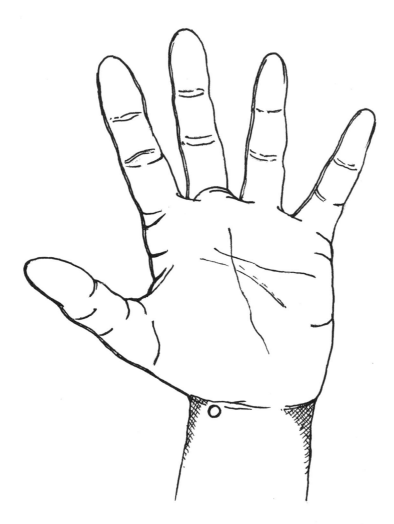

LU 9 (Lung Channel)

On the palm side of the transverse wrist crease, in the depression beneath the thumb, between the point where you can feel your radial pulse and the tendon that goes to your thumb, is the location of LU9.

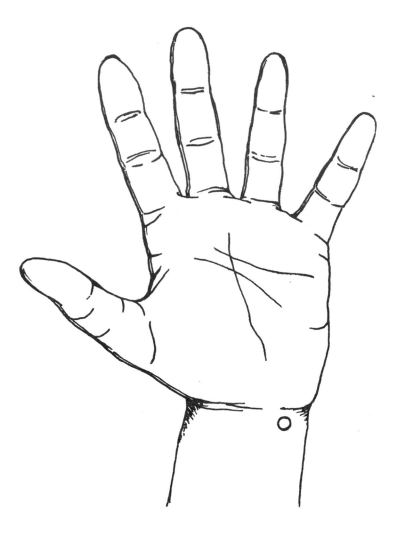

HT7 (Heart Channel)

Start at the underside of the wrist at the end of the ulna bone (outer wrist bone) by the transverse crease of the wrist. The point is located in the depression on the radial side of the tendon of the flexor carpi ulnaris muscle.

Smell: Herbs, Flowers, Plants, and Essential Oils*—Ginger and Peppermint

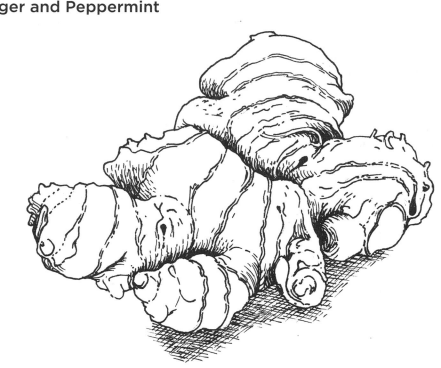

Ginger (*Zingiber officinale*)

Ginger is one of the most ancient spices used for medicinal purposes. Its wide-ranging uses are reflected in its Sanskrit name, which means "universal medicine." For teens dealing with withdrawal or similar symptoms, it has two very useful qualities. First, it can alleviate certain kinds of nausea. Second, it has been associated with having anti-inflammatory properties and research has supported gastro-intestinal benefits. (Takahashi et al., 2010; Pillai et al., 2011; Weimer et al., 2012)

*Essential Oils (EO) have several methods of use. Please refer to the Treatment Protocol Information and Resource Guide of this book (page 197) for additional detailed information on aromatherapy.

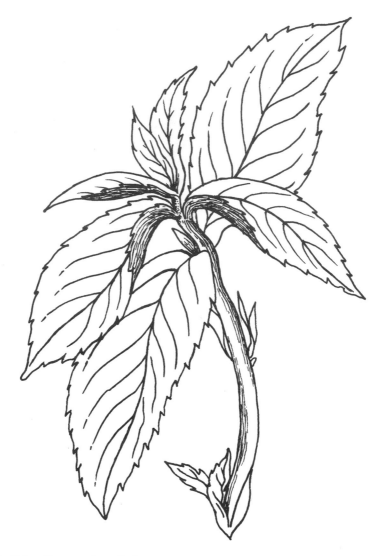

Peppermint (*Mentha × piperita*)

This herb can assist with opening up congested sinuses, help ease coughing related to congestion, and support the respiratory system's ability to function optimally. Peppermint essential oil has traditionally been used to help ease labored breathing (for example, as seen in the process of smoking cessation) and has also been linked with relaxation of the mind and digestion. This helps both headache and stomach upset, which are common when quitting substances of abuse. This added support can increase a sense of well-being that can help teens maintain their commitment and resolve to combat cravings associated with withdrawal.

Taste: Herbal Tisanes*—Siberian Ginseng, Passionflower, Dandelion, Thyme

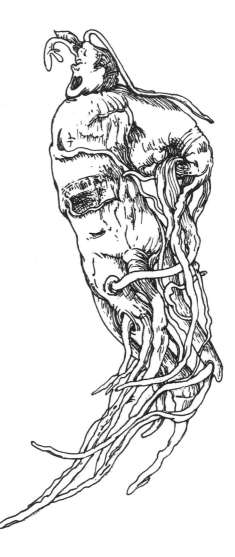

Siberian Ginseng

(*Eleutherococcus senticosus*)

Siberian ginseng comes from a shrub in the Far East, ranging from 3 to 10 feet in height. The root of the plant is used for treatments. It can be easily consumed as a solid or in a dried version for tea. It has a tangy taste that is reminiscent of ginger. One of its main chemicals, eleutheroside, may be able to reduce the stress response in humans by reducing activity in the adrenal cortex. Siberian ginseng is known for an ability to counteract lack of appetite and insomnia, two conditions that can affect people going through withdrawal.

*Tea and herbal tisanes are easy to prepare and find at local stores and markets. For detailed information on preparation and sourcing please refer to the Treatment Protocol Information and Resource Guide on page 197.

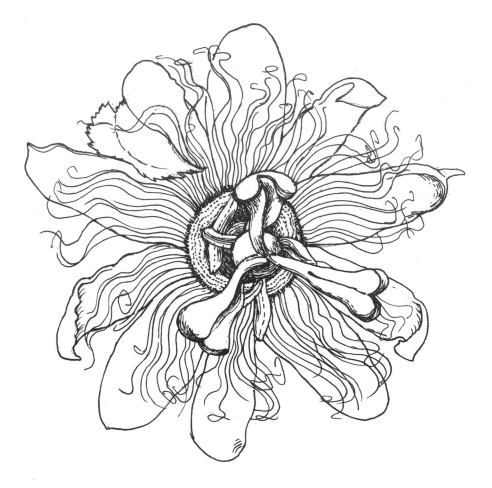

Passionflower (*Passiflora incarnata*)

This very flamboyant flower can be several inches across, in contrasting colors of purple and white. It originated in tropical and subtropical parts of the western hemisphere and was traditionally used in the Americas, then spread to Europe. It's most often administered as an infusion of the dried flowers in water. Research has shown beneficial effects on anxiety and insomnia. Due to passionflower's calming and sedating properties, one study highlighted its ability to aid in opiate withdrawal symptoms. Also, used in combination with drugs that deal with withdrawal symptoms, such as irritability, it seems to enhance the effectiveness of those drugs. (Miyasaka et al., 2007; Akhondzadeh et al., 2001)

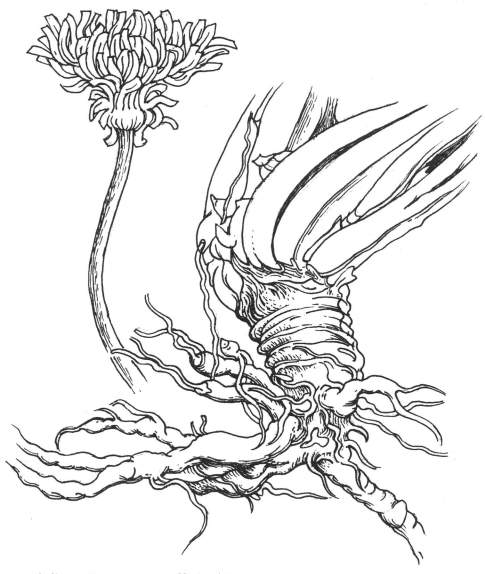

Dandelion (*Taraxacum officinale*)

The English name comes from the Latin *dens leonis*, which means "lion's teeth." It's been used for centuries and can be consumed in a variety of ways, eaten in salad or brewed in a tea. It's known for its great detoxifying powers and *in vitro* studies have linked this herb with the suppression of cancer cells. (Jang, 2011; Menghini, 2010)

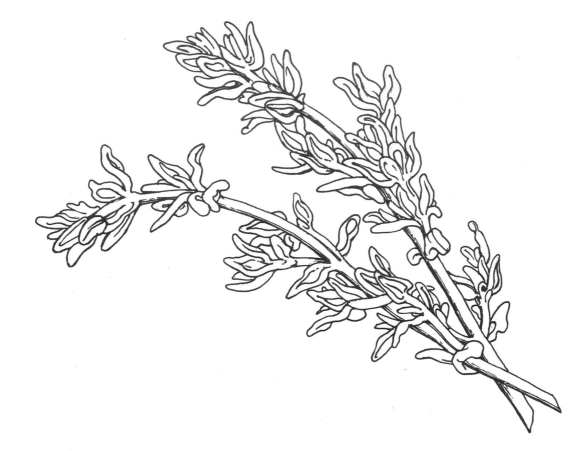

Thyme (*Thymus vulgaris*)

Wild thyme grows in southern Europe but is now cultivated worldwide. It has great antiseptic and tonic qualities. It grows as a diminutive evergreen shrub with a lemony scent and is a great complement to many popular dishes. Thyme is reported to help with alcoholism—both in reducing cravings and in helping to repair damage to the liver (in animal models). (Rašković, et al., 2015)

Sight: Yoga Postures—Happy Baby, Child's Pose, Sitting Mountain

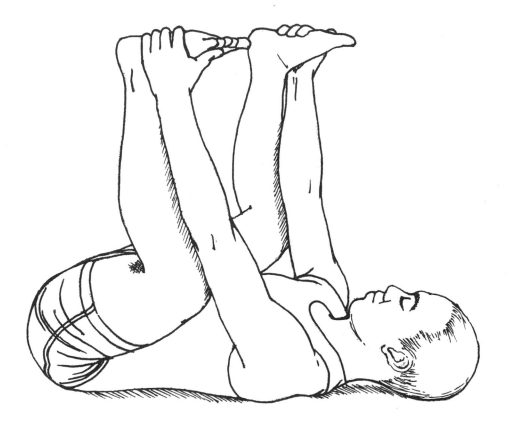

Happy Baby

For this pose, just imagine yourself as a baby, putting your legs up in the air and grabbing your toes. With your hands grabbing at the outside of your feet, the stretches are achieved by pushing your feet up and pulling your hands down at the same time. If it's difficult to grab your feet with your hands, use a strap of some sort around the feet.

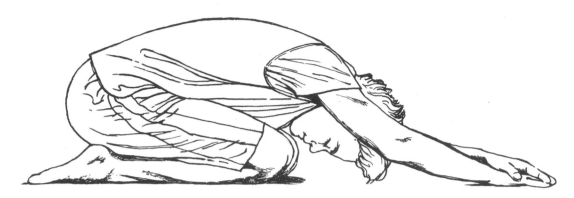

Child's Pose

As described in Chapter 2, Child's Pose is very restorative and may help ameliorate some of the withdrawal and anxiety symptoms that sometimes accompany attempts to stop a substance abuse habit.

Sitting Mountain

This is a seated pose, as the title implies. In addition to sitting, the arms are engaged by interlacing the fingers and then stretching the arms above the head. This should be done during the exhale breath. This calms the body and relaxes the mind. Once arms are stretched they can be returned palms down with one hand resting on each thigh as shown in the illustration. These are both excellent preparations for meditation, which can be a useful tool in restraining the cravings of a person suffering from substance abuse.

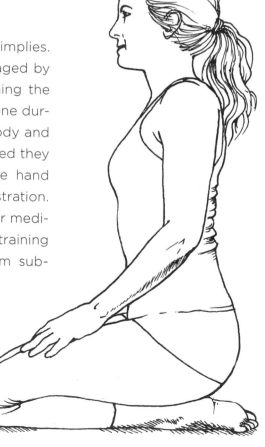

Sound: Relaxing, Harmonic music, Meditative Sounds

People dealing with substance abuse often respond best to therapy regimens that employ many different approaches, with music being one possible avenue of therapy. Music that promotes and assists with guided muscle relaxation (relaxing, harmonic music or balanced aligned sounds) can be very helpful. Isochronic beats have been found to temporarily alter brainwave patterns and may help those dealing with substance abuse to change their habits and thought patterns related to substance abuse. Isochronic tones are beats that are turned on and off rapidly, creating a sharp sound pulse. In one study, a scientist created four very different activities around music: a music guessing game, lyric analysis, guided imagery, and songwriting. Although patients in the study had no strong preference for any particular intervention, all were enthusiastic about music therapy and noted that it had a strong positive impact on them (Silverman, 2003).

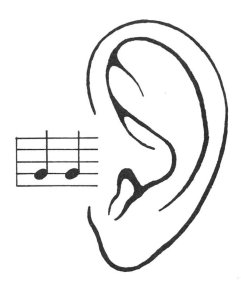

Conclusion:
CAM and the Science So Far

COMPLEMENTARY AND ALTERNATIVE medicine (CAM) can be placed in four broad categories, as defined by the National Institutes of Health: (1) mind-body intervention, (2) biologically based therapies (diet, supplements, and herbs), (3) manipulation and body-based therapies, and (4) energy therapies (acupuncture, Reiki, magnets, therapeutic touch, and others; Gaylord & Mann, 2007). But CAM really encompasses a dizzying variety of new and old approaches to health interventions. For people in the West, they might be better understood by what they are not: "They are outside [the] mainstream U.S. health care paradigm, with its emphasis on pharmaceuticals, surgery, biotechnology, controlled clinical trials, and traditional scientific methods" (Gaylord & Mann, 2007).

Options from outside the "U.S. health care paradigm" are not new. Midwives, for instance, who were also purveyors of a wide variety of folk remedies for centuries, encountered resistance from university-trained male doctors armed with their professional credentials starting in the mid-eighteenth century (Ulrich, 1990). In the late nineteenth century, William James—philosopher, psychologist, scientist, and MD—railed against the Massachusetts medical profession for supporting a law that would, in essence, outlaw alternative therapies for mental health ailments. In 1894, James wrote to the *Boston Evening Transcript*:

The suppression of certain practitioners will hinder the progress of therapeutic knowledge as a whole. And, to be concrete, I will confine myself to a class of diseases with which my occupation has made me somewhat conversant. I mean diseases of the nervous system and the mind. . . .

The gain to science [in neurology] has been almost exclusively in the way of anatomy, symptoms, classification and diagnosis; and the hypnotics, anaesthetics, sedatives and stimulants of various sorts discovered [through science], although brilliantly effective over momentary states, bear little relation to the patient's permanent cure. . . .

I assuredly hold no brief for any of these [mind] healers, and must confess that my intellect has been unable to assimilate their theories, so far as I have heard them given. But their *facts* are patent and startling; and anything that interferes with the multiplication of such facts, and with our freest opportunity of observing and studying them, will, I believe, be a public calamity. (James, 1987)

James would certainly be supportive of today's doctors who, like himself, were impressed with the positive reports of CAM therapies and, because of those results, wanted to learn more about them.

In the last 15 years, many of the barriers that have separated CAM therapies from traditional scientific health care have begun to come down. One of the most notable changes is the interest by the U.S. government's National Institutes of Health in seriously studying CAM (through the National Center for Complementary and Integrative Health, or NCCIH, formerly called the National Center for Complementary and Alternative Medicine, or NCCAM). Moreover, in the early 2000s, NCCAM began funding "15 projects [that] were designed to incorporate CAM information into the curricula of conventional health professions schools" (Gaylord & Mann, 2007; see also Pearson & Chesney, 2007). The maximum grant was $300,000 a year for a maximum of 5 years, for a total investment of $22.5 million. All of the recipients were accredited and reputable academic centers, which were joined by some prestigious institutions, such as Children's Hospital, Boston. What explains this about-face in which conventionally scientific institutions have not only ceased their assault against CAM, but have actually made efforts to integrate CAM into more conventional medicine?

The prime impetus for this change came not from doctors but their patients.

While an explanation of the cultural reasons behind this increase in the popularity of CAM is beyond the bounds of this book, the raw numbers describing the growth of CAM in the general population begin to explain why conventional medicine began to take these therapies seriously.

For instance, between 1990 and 1997, visits to alternative practitioners soared from 470 million to 629 million. (In contrast, in 1997 there were 386 million visits to primary care physicians in the United States.) In terms of resources, that translated into $27 billion in out-of-pocket expenses paid by patients for CAM therapies. And in 1998, 42% of adults surveyed reported using CAM therapies (Gaylord & Mann, 2007).

Doctors all over the United States discovered that their patients were adopting CAM therapies, because the patients clearly thought they would have some impact on their health. More alarmingly, despite these trends, doctors were also finding that their patients were reluctant to share information about the CAM treatments they had adopted. The reasons ranged from not believing it was the doctor's business to fearing that a conventional doctor would disapprove or discourage the application of CAM therapies (Gaylord & Mann, 2007).

A profound medical and cultural disconnect, then, was beginning to widen the distance between doctors and patients. It was bad enough that doctors were often unaware of treatments that would have an impact on a patient's well-being. What was potentially worse was a gulf of trust between doctor and patient, one in which silence about CAM treatments could grow into suspicion of a doctor's medical advice to the patient. So, for medical and cultural reasons, integrating CAM into the mainstream curricula—normalizing it as a possible source of healing—began in the early 2000s.

While the need for doctors to familiarize themselves with CAM was obvious, what to do with the new information was less obvious. The main problem deterring many doctors from embracing CAM or applying it to many different patients was the lack of data on its applicability and efficiency for a wide variety of patient needs and in a wide variety of contexts. That data, though sometimes sparse, is now beginning to accumulate.

Before doctors can have confidence in prescribing an alternative technique to their patients, they must be convinced that there is not only safety, but also efficacy, or effectiveness, in these new approaches. Indeed, no scientist or doctor would prescribe a course of treatment based on word of mouth or anecdotal experiences alone. The public would never be served if they did. That is why so many patients who, in the past, had asked their doctor for their opinion on alternative treatments often heard the response: "You can try it, but there's no evidence that it works."

But this knowledge base is changing. The fact that we now have a federally funded division of the NIH studying the question of what works is significant. It means that evidence-based research is now becoming available to the medical profession and to the public. In addition, there are now at least 69 peer-reviewed scientific journals that publish CAM-related research (Morgan, Littman, Palmer, Singh, & LaRiccia, 2012).

Because so many alternative interventions are free or low cost (think of meditation and yoga), proving efficacy logically means that people might be healed at a lower overall cost to society, and at a lower cost to health insurance companies. Currently, NCCIH does not advocate replacing medical treatment with CAM, but advises them to be used together synergistically. Hence the words "complementary" and "integrative" always appear in the collective name. It's clear that the ramifications of CAM's adoption into mainstream medicine has multifaceted benefits.

Since 1999, NCCIH has funded or partially funded more than 1,500 studies, including studies of herbal supplements and physical interventions. That's a lot of research to inform the public on the usefulness of particular therapies, and one reason why more and more mainstream doctors are beginning to suggest things like meditation for their patients with anxiety, or yoga for back pain sufferers, for example. The value of having an independent entity funding the studies means that both positive and negative results are of equal importance because there is no fundamental conflict of interest, or potential for monetary gain.

An important concept to keep in mind when educating oneself on the CAM literature is that not all studies are equal or hold the same weight. This is true in all scientific research. For example, a study that enrolls 25 subjects cannot be as confident in its conclusions as a similar study that enrolls 500. Also, a study that relies on self-reporting—that is, subjects asked to fill out questionnaires about their experiences—is considered less reliable than, say, a study that involves measuring heart rate and blood pressure. In the first case, any improvements reported from the treatment are subjective, while in the second case, the outcome data are objective and measurable by any medical professional. Finally, CAM research, like most medical research, uses adults as subjects. Since adolescents are young adults, outcomes are assumed to be relevant to the teenage patient population as well, even though the teenage brain is quite dynamic and unique, as described earlier. However, there are very few studies of CAM approaches for adolescents per se.

A summary of 16 years of CAM research can be described thus: There is undeniable evidence that some, but not all, CAM treatments show efficacy and promise, and are worthy of further research. When a small study with, say, 50 subjects shows efficacy, it paves the way for potential funding for a larger study.

Let's take a look at the latest research related to the treatments we use in our clinic.

ESSENTIAL OILS

Although there are far too many essential oils to analyze here, for the sake of our review, I will consider lavender. It may be one of the most studied of the essential oils. Lavender's legendary soothing and sedative properties have been well documented overseas, particularly in South Korea and Germany, where even tea made from the lavender flower is approved for use in insomnia, restlessness, and stomach irritation (Lavender, 2015). Numerous studies have shown that it promotes a calm state of mind and mildly induces a sleep state. So lavender is a good choice for stress reduction overall. It clearly promotes a calmer mind and improved sense of well-being, and it seems to take the edge off stress, pain, and agitation. One fascinating study from 2006 involving 50 women who had just undergone breast biopsy surgery, showed that lavender was effective in helping them with postoperative pain (Kim et al., 2006).

U.S. research on lavender has been sparse overall. And there's always the odd study that shows no effect. For example, one protocol in which subjects were "stressed" by peeling tape off their skin or immersing their feet in ice water showed no pain mitigation effects from lavender (Kiecolt-Glaser et al., 2008). Of course one can argue that the stress triggers in this case barely resemble the real-life symptoms that would indicate lavender use. Nevertheless, practitioners need to consider the whole body of research on a particular approach to evaluate its benefit. Further, other essential oils such as lemon and rosemary have also been associated with health benefits. A host of additional essential oils have been studied and appear in international research journals. But myriad oils used in aromatherapy have yet to be studied scientifically.

YOGA

One of the top 10 complementary therapies, yoga is sought out for health issues by about 6% of adults (National Center for Complementary and Integrative Health, 2013). With a long tradition in Indian culture, yoga combines stretching, strength poses, and relaxation to enhance and create a deep sense of well-being. Much like regular exercise, ongoing yoga practice can help ease symptoms of depression, insomnia, and anxiety.

In the clinical realm, some large studies have shown that yoga practice improves chronic back pain more effectively than conventional medical treatment. (A stretching routine also gets similar high marks; National Center for Complementary and Integrative Health, 2013.) But the studies that look at yoga's impact on health problems such as asthma and arthritis show no conclusive benefit (National Center for Complementary and Integrative Health, 2013). Many more protocols are underway that look at yoga's impact on menopause, smoking cessation, and diabetes, to name a few. Its growing popularity indicates that many people are turning to yoga to improve their lifestyle, fitness, and well-being—not necessarily because they have specific medical problems. One can assume that staying flexible and balanced through the aging process can only help with physical and emotional resilience.

ACUPUNCTURE

Practiced for thousands of years in many Asian cultures, and an integral component of Chinese medicine, acupuncture is perhaps the most controversial of alternative therapies currently under study. More than 3,000 trials of acupuncture have been conducted over several decades. A robust debate has emerged about acupuncture's usefulness. A vocal group of doctors believe that, taken as a whole, the research results show that acupuncture is little more effective than a placebo and therefore does not meet Western medicine's standards of efficacy (Colquhoun & Novella, 2013). They believe doctors should not prescribe or suggest this treatment to patients so that they do not waste their money and time on an intervention that does not work.

This is a powerful statement to make about such a globally embraced treatment, one for which so many users report health benefits. The most powerful evidence in acupuncture's favor are the many current studies that show acupuncture is effective in treating chronic back, knee, and neck pain. In 2003, the World Health Organization, after synthesizing thousands of results from controlled clinical trials, concluded that acupuncture was effective (not just safe) in treating more than 40 conditions, from depression and nausea to stroke and rheumatoid arthritis.

So what accounts for the controversy? Like many studies in the area of alternative medicine, acupuncture outcomes depend on self-reporting. So, patients report subjectively on whether or not their symptoms have improved. Often this is done by rating the severity of their symptoms on a scale of, say, 1 to 10, before and after the treatment. (In a controlled clinical trial, of course, there will be a control group that gets a sham treatment, or no intervention at all, that is, the placebo.) When a study shows that the treatment group reports slightly more improvement than a placebo group, it becomes tricky to draw conclusions. The authors of the study then have to decide how to characterize the result—is acupuncture about as good as a placebo (and therefore not effective), or is it better than a placebo and therefore effective? And how much better than a placebo does it have to be to be declared effective? There are no hard and fast rules about how to interpret two sets of data that are not very far apart. And this is the essence of the controversy: Most studies that deem acupuncture to be effective have outcomes that are better—but only slightly better—than a placebo. So how to interpret this gray area? In my opinion, and in the opinion of many other researchers, the slight advantage over placebo, combined with a wealth of positive anecdotal and clinical outcomes, puts acupuncture on safe ground as an effective, evidence-based treatment for a variety of conditions. This balance of evidence has now paved the way for integrating acupuncture into Western medicine. The newer laser and electronic acupuncture treatments are also reporting the same stress and pain relief outcomes as needles (Law, Baxter, & Tumilty, 2015).

Self-reporting is not the only way to measure the benefits of acupuncture. An empirical method of measuring the impact of a treatment is by looking at the physiological changes that occur as a result of the treatment. For example, studies have tracked the reduction of stress-related hormones in the body, and others use brain imaging to see what areas are affected during treatment and if they correspond to known regions for pain or stress reduction.

A study conducted at the Georgetown University School of Nursing found that rats that were experimentally stressed could be brought back to homeostasis via electronic acupuncture applied to a point on the knee. The researchers measured blood hormone levels secreted by the hypothalamus, the pituitary gland, and the adrenal gland known as the hypothalamic-pituitary-adrenal (HPA) axis. They also measured a protein involved in the animals' fight-or-flight response, called NPY. Their conclusion: "electronic acupuncture blocks the chronic, stress-induced elevations of the HPA axis hormones and the sympathetic NPY pathway" (Eshkevari, et al., 2003). This exciting finding indicates a biological response at the molecular level, and one that scientists may want to attempt to replicate in humans.

Finally, neuroimaging studies reveal that acupuncture modulates a wide network of brain regions, including areas related to pain, attention, higher cognition, and the autonomous nervous system (Dhond, Kettner, & Napadow, 2007). How these regions correspond to specific acupoints is a potentially rich vein of investigation.

ACUPRESSURE

Although not studied as extensively as acupuncture, self-administered acupressure is gaining interest among researchers. Instead of using fine needles, points in the body are stimulated using pressure applied for several minutes, most often by the thumb and forefinger. The point on the wrist called P6 has been well studied and shown to effectively reduce nausea in a variety of conditions, including pregnancy and chemotherapy treatment. The positive effect on nausea has also been recorded in children (Susan G. Komen, 2015). Many are familiar with the wristbands worn to reduce the nausea from seasickness; the protrusions on the bracelet apply pressure to the P6 point. Other studies show that acupressure can improve cognitive function in patients with mild traumatic brain injury, and also reduce anxiety (McFadden et al., 2011).

Because it is one of the most convenient, quick, and cost-free approaches to self-care, I believe acupressure has the potential to gain wide acceptance among the adolescent population. Not only does it give teens an independent mode for addressing their symptoms, but also it appeals to parents who would like to try any and all noninvasive interventions for their child, before a small symptom, such as anxiety, escalates into a serious disorder.

SOUND AND MUSIC THERAPY

The value of music therapy in the treatment of brain injury is well documented. Music therapy is widespread in rehabilitation settings worldwide, where it is used to help restore speech and other cognitive functions for people with brain trauma and injury, and it has been shown to reduce anxiety and depression in people suffering from Alzheimer's disease. Newer applications include therapy for ADHD and autism. This method of therapy was in the spotlight several years ago with the story of the attack on Arizona congresswoman Gabrielle Giffords, who was shot in the left temple, injuring the speech region of her brain. In her long recovery process, Giffords used music therapy to help her right brain learn how to talk again by singing words before she spoke them.

The mode of therapy can be music or individual sounds. Music is a complex and structured arrangement of sounds, and it is hypothesized that it can help to organize or calm the mind. Individual sounds may theoretically be able to interrupt repetitive or perseverative thought patterns in people with anxiety and depression.

Music has been shown to decrease stress hormone (cortisol) levels in depressed adolescents (Field et al., 1998). Music is often a constant companion to teenagers, and it's a powerful way to connect their thoughts and emotions to something pleasurable. That is why it's a go-to therapy for young clients, and one that is increasingly having a positive impact. For example, a large randomized controlled trial in Northern Ireland that looked at 250 depressed and anxious teenagers found significant increases in self-esteem and reduced depression after a treatment plan that included music for relaxation, songwriting, and improvisation (Porter et al., 2012).

In our clinical setting, we encouraged our clients to use music to take a mental break from their troubling thoughts, or to use it preemptively to focus the mind in anticipation of a known stressor. Being able to return to a baseline of pleasure or calm is a powerful self-regulating habit. Research is just beginning to show music's long-term benefit in treating anxiety and depression. However, there are numerous ways to design and apply music and sound in therapy, so more specificity will be needed in future studies to determine the value of each approach.

TEA AND HERBAL TISANES

Tea drinking has recently become more popular among teens and young adults, and this trend can be seen in the proliferation of tea bars or cafés that specialize in brewed teas. It is not uncommon for adolescents in urban areas to meet up with friends at a tea bar, in much the same way that adults might meet a friend for a drink in a pub. This renewed interest in tea makes it easy for my clients to adopt tea drinking as a regular part of their day: It's not just for grandma any-more—tea drinking has become downright cool. In addition to being naturally calorie free, tea contributes to total water intake, so it can benefit the kids who don't hydrate often enough.

Tea offers a wide variety of health benefits; let's discuss some of them here. Tea is a major source of dietary flavonoids, which appear to affect health in a variety of ways, such as providing cardiovascular and cognitive benefits. But it's in the area of heart health that some of the strongest evidence exists in support of tea's value for wellness. Many observational studies, several clinical trials, and systematic reviews and meta-analyses have found an association between tea consumption and reduced risk of heart disease and stroke. Tea consumption might lower the risk of stroke or mortality by improving nitric oxide synthesis or reducing nitric oxide breakdown, thus linking tea and reduced risk of cardiovascular events and stroke (U.S. Department of Agriculture and U.S. Department of Health and Human Services, 2010).

Inverse associations between tea consumption and cancer risk have been observed in large, prospective cohort studies, especially for esophageal, gastric, rectal, and colon cancers, findings consistent with an extensive body of experimental evidence (Vinson, Teufel, & Wu, 2004; Balentine, Wiserman, & Bouwens, 1997; Geleijnse, Launer, Van der Kuip, Hofman, & Witteman, 2002). Tea affords cognitive benefits. Tea polyphenols are bioavailable to the brain and effect neuroprotective or neuro-rescue actions in cell cultures and animal models (Mandel,

Amit, Kalfon, Reznichenko, & Youdim, 2008; Rezai-Zadeh et al., 2005). And this is not to mention the perceived effect tea has on mood, cognitive functioning, and alertness.

Tea plays a role in weight management. Catechin- and caffeine-rich teas (CCRTs), such as green, oolong, and white tea, have been proposed to maintain or enhance energy expenditure and to increase fat oxidation. Research related to CCRTs demonstrates improvements in body weight, body mass index, body fat mass, and waist-to-hip ratio in studies and meta-analyses (Balentine et al., 1997).

Of late, green tea studies have captured most of the media attention, but there is evidence for health support from both green and black teas. A number of studies have supported black tea and cardiovascular health. One study found as little as one cup per day for 3 weeks showed improved cholesterol values (with approximately 10% decrease in LDL; Vinson et al., 2004). Researchers aren't sure why green or black tea reduces the risk of heart disease by lowering cholesterol and triglyceride levels. Further research is needed to better define the relationship between tea consumption and potential benefit to lipid profiles. Yet it is promising that some studies estimate black tea to decrease the rate of heart attack by 11% with consumption of three cups of tea per day (Deka & Vita, 2011; Peters, Poole, & Arab, 2001).

Another study out of University College in London showed that tea drinkers (several cups per day, with a minimum of two) were able to recover from the effects of stress more quickly than those who drank a tea substitute (Steptoe et al., 2007). Studies support that black tea can lower blood platelet activation, which is linked to blood clotting, heart attack, and stroke. It can support thinning the blood and play a role in decreasing the risk of certain cardiovascular conditions.

Furthermore, tea offers protective benefit against diabetes. A 2012 European study found tea to be an effective way to reduce the risk of developing type 2 diabetes. In countries where citizens drank four or more cups per day, they had a 20% lower risk of developing the illness (Striege, Kang, Pilkenton, Rychlik, & Apostolidis, 2015). The benefit is believed to be associated with glucose digestion and uptake.

One important compound specific to tea definitely helps to relax and induce a sense of calm, which is L-theanine. It's an amino acid present almost exclusively in tea that produces a calming effect on the brain.

Japanese researchers discovered that theanine is a caffeine antagonist, offsetting the stimulating or antsy, jittery effect of caffeine but allowing improved attention and mental performance (Nobre, Rao, & Owen, 2008). So there is a synergistic effect with theanine and caffeine. Incidentally, of the 20 different types of amino acids in tea, more than 60% are theanine. Also, to best appreciate what is happening in the body during periods of stress, it's important to look at what occurs during the stress response. We are hardwired to respond quickly and fully to a given stress or perceived threat. What gets triggered at that time is the fight-or-flight hormone cortisol, which causes a cascade of physiological changes, so your body can react to the threat and then return to a calm baseline state we call homeostasis. But we live in a constant overstimulated state where we are overworked, overtired, eating poorly on the go, and we get depleted. This is a perpetual state of stress in the body. One of the ways our bodies respond is by activating inflammatory pathways and producing inflammation. In medicine, we are learning more and more about how chronic inflammatory states can be detrimental to our health.

Other compounds in tea separate from theanine that promote mental relaxation are the catechins, a type of polyphenols which are under the broader category of antioxidants. But the main consensus at this point is that the health benefits of these compounds are not due to their ability to act as classic antioxidants (i.e., extinguishing free radicals that cause cell damage—cancer). Rather, they act on biomarkers of inflammation to modulate a host of cell signal transduction pathways. Some of these actions result in the upregulation of antioxidant enzymes (e.g., catalase, GSHPx, SOD) and thus of antioxidant defenses. Therefore catechins exert a supporting role in helping to control or diminish the inflammatory responses in our body that can lead to numerous negative health consequences if left unchecked over time.

As a final point of interest, true teas come from one plant, *Camellia sinensis*. So infusing the parts of this plant makes tea. Any other herbs infused, brewed, or steeped make a tisane, which is a French word meaning "infusion or decoction." Some commonly used tisanes include chamomile, rosehips, peppermint or lemongrass—of course, there are many others. The health benefits of herbal tisanes are vast and varied. Research in this area continues to grow.

WHAT IF IT'S ALL JUST A PLACEBO?

As noted above, perhaps tens of thousands of studies have been conducted on alternative therapies ranging from vitamin supplements to yoga. Many show that an intervention is effective, but whether or not it's effective enough to enter mainstream clinical settings is the question under debate. A growing number of medical doctors such as myself believe that enough empirical evidence exists for the interventions discussed in this book to justify their adoption as a complement to mainstream Western medicine.

In fact, some alternative therapies have already entered the mainstream. In the United States, most private and public health insurance plans offer some coverage for chiropractic care and massage, although the number of visits and extent of coverage are limited. Does this mean that only insurance-approved interventions work and we should abandon the others? No, it simply means the medical establishment is in the process of catching up to recent research on a variety of interventions.

Medical research may also need to embrace a new method for assessing outcomes in terms of lifestyle improvement, increases in well-being, and behavior change, criteria that pose a challenge to measure, but ones that will inevitably lead to better long-term health. In addition to looking for objective clinical data such as blood pressure reduction or stress hormones in the blood, which one might find, for example, in a randomized controlled trial (RCT), there is a compelling argument for relying more on patient-reported outcomes (PROs) in the evaluation of holistic therapies. As one team of anthropologists explains:

> Given the fact that most CAM use is for health promotion (Davis et al., 2011a), and that much of treatment-oriented CAM is aimed at chronic pain and mood disorders (Barnes et al., 2008), PROs are likely better measures of the "real world" clinical goals of CAM therapies than are RCTs. Anthropologists are involved in developing PRO measures that look beyond presenting symptoms and specific treatment objectives to capture multi-dimensional shifts in well-being following CAM therapies (Ritenbaugh et al., under review; Thompson et al., under review). (Thompson & Nichter, 2011)

But let's consider the current, conventional belief that CAM therapies offer only a slight improvement over a placebo in controlled clinical trials. (Certainly some studies show a stronger difference than this characterization.) I posit that even a slightly improved outcome, as captured in a study, can translate into great improvements in health and well-being over time via behavior change and adoption of self-care skills. Interestingly, in economic terms, even slight improvements in health can translate into lower health care costs. Evidence is starting to emerge that patients with certain conditions who use CAM have lower insurance expenditures than those who use only conventional care, by incurring fewer inpatient stays and imaging diagnostics (Lind, Lafferty, Tyree, & Diehr, 2010).

So a strong case can be made that alternative therapies have the potential to be a cost-effective strategy for insurance companies. Considering that chronic disease is the leading cause of death and disability in the United States, costing us $277 billion per year (DeVol & Bedroussian, 2007), and also taking into account the low cost of many alternative therapies, it seems logical that CAM therapies should be more widely offered and affordable to everyone. (While alternative medicine accounts for only about 1.5% of total health care spending in the United States, it is 11.2% of total out-of-pocket health care spending, according to the 2007 National Health Interview Survey.)

The economic argument is, perhaps, not the most compelling one for the widespread adoption of CAM. Instead, it is the wealth of evidence flowing from clinical experience that drives the momentum for more holistic and noninvasive healing options. Watching my teenage patients improve, and witnessing their power to take control of their mental health, is a testament to the profound health benefits that CAM offers to this adolescent population. The measure of success, in my mind, is not only when a teenager responds to therapy by getting back on track with her energy, focus, and ability to have fun, but also when she effusively tells her story of health improvement to her peers. But perhaps the most affirmative outcome is finding out, years later, that she still turns to her toolbox of interventions for help when handling the setbacks and challenges of life. It is this resilience that underpins the hope and promise of alternative therapies.

Sensory Treatment Protocol Information and Resource Guide

//

SENSORY TREATMENT PROTOCOL INFORMATION:

TOUCH—Acupressure Points

As described in the various "Touch" sections of each protocol, the acupressure points can be easily stimulated and massaged. It's important to note that most acupressure (and acupuncture) points located on the limbs (arms and legs) are bilateral. By convention, only one limb acupressure point is shown, but bilateral stimulation is the goal. Each point can be activated separately. For example, if a point on the arm or wrist is shown, first activate the acupressure point on one arm (right or left) and then, once that treatment is completed activate the acupressure point on the opposite limb.

SMELL—Herbs, Flowers, Plants, and Essential Oils

There are many ways to use essential oils (EOs). For aromatherapy, you can place several drops of the EO on a tissue or gauze and hold near your nostrils for approximately two minutes while you inhale deeply and exhale slowly and gently. EOs can also be placed in a diffuser (the device combines EO and water blends) for more long-term room dispersion. For use with a diffuser, follow packaging instructions for individual device use. Finally, you can place them topically on pulse points (wrists, neck, and temples).

Should you want to apply an EO topically, blend the EO in a carrier oil or water (for spray or aerosol form) before application. EOs are highly concentrated plant essences. Some of these oils when applied on their own can irritate skin and are best combined with a carrier oil such as jojoba, coconut, grapeseed, or wheat germ. There are many others. Almond oil is another option but for those with a nut allergy is it best to avoid it and use a different carrier oil.

When applied topically, you only need a few drops of the EO added to the carrier oil, and briefly massage gently over the area to aid absorption. Typically, use 6–12 drops of the EO to one ounce of the carrier oil. Depending on individual sensitivity, you can adjust using less EO per ounce of carrier oil.

Another form of application is an atomizer or air spritzer/spray. Use approximately 10–15 drops of EO per one ounce of water. Shake well before spraying.

TASTE: Tea and Herbal Tisanes

To prepare tea: For green tea (as mentioned in Chapter 7 as a sensory treatment for focus and concentration) water should be heated to approx. 175–185 degrees. Add 1 teaspoon or one tea bag for 8 ounces of water. Once tea is added to hot water steep time is 1–3 minutes. Steep times can vary depending on taste preference. The tea will have a stronger taste is you steep for a longer period of time. If you steep for too long, the tea can take on a bitter taste.

Should you have an interest in trying other teas, here is a general guide: white teas use approximately the same water temperature (175–185 degrees) and steep time as green tea. There are always slight variations depending on the specific tea. Black teas are best prepared using a higher water temperature 200–205 degrees and a steep time of 3–5 minutes.

Herbal tisanes, as provided in treatment protocol sections for Chapters 2–8, require a higher water temperature for preparation than teas. Typically, 200–210 degrees. The steep time is also longer, with 5 or 5+ minutes for best extraction of the tisanes flavors and health compounds. Many herbs are more robust plants than the tea (*Camellia sinensis*) plant. For that reason, they tend to need more time infused in water for optimal extraction.

As you become more familiar with tea and herbal tisanes you can prepare them with certain variations that are specific to your own taste. Both the preparation and use of these healthy beverages should be enjoyable and provide a type of meditative or ritual practice to your daily routine.

SIGHT: Yoga Postures

There are many different yoga positions or postures mentioned in this book. For each yoga pose provided at the end of Chapters 2–8 (Treatment Protocol Sections), once you follow the instruction for that particular pose you should ensure that you are not in discomfort, and holding any of the poses should not cause pain.

Once you are comfortably in a pose, hold that position for 1–5 minutes while breathing slowly and deeply. Neither your inhalations nor your exhalations should be quick and shallow. Proper breathing during yoga practice is an integral part of reaping the greatest benefit from the treatment. Make sure you don't hold your breath. While there is a range of breathing used in yoga practice, slowing your breaths to 6–10 per minute is a good place to start. Keep in mind that the average person has a respiratory rate of 12–20 breaths per minute. Use that as a guide and adjust as your comfort level allows.

In terms of how long to hold a pose, there is some variation. This depends on your ease and readiness to assume the various poses. You can also decide whether you want to hold a position (static pose) or combine it with other poses into movements (dynamic poses). Make the program your own and add duration to each pose and couple different poses into a series as you gain mastery of the different treatment protocols provided in Chapters 2-8.

If you have any medical conditions or injuries that may prevent you from attempting some of the poses depicted in this book please check with your healthcare provider to ensure you can safely engage in the physical postures without causing further injury or risk.

SOUND: Sound and Music Therapy

As discussed in each chapter's Treatment Protocol section, the sounds and types of music that can be utilized are vast. We offer general guidance as to the basic types that can be helpful for certain conditions. How these sounds are to be enjoyed can vary as well. You can use a personal device such as a smart phone with earbuds for an individual listening experience. Another option is to play these sounds, songs, or soundtracks on a freestanding device with a speaker that fills the room. This is part of the individualized nature of these holistic treatments that the user can choose and tailor their desired experience.

This also applies to the type of music you choose to listen to. While we provide descriptions of the tempos, beats, sounds, and other qualities that best target a given condition and may provide relief, the ultimate choice within that range can be individualized to best resonate with the user. For example, in Chapter 3 we discuss fatigue. For this condition, we suggest that "steady, upbeat [tempo], and positive-sounding music" can improve your sense of well-being. In that range, one might choose, as some patients have, Aerosmith's "Sweet Emotion" while others prefer Michael Jackson's "Don't Stop 'Til You Get Enough." Again, there is room to design a tailored playlist of sounds and music that best suit and are pleasurable to the listener.

The duration of the sound and music therapy can also vary. For some, 5–10 minutes of targeted listening may be sufficient. If your setting or particular circumstance allows, more time can be devoted to listening. Again, this is a personal journey that allows you some latitude in creating the best individualized treatment protocol.

RESOURCE GUIDE:

TOUCH: Acupressure and Acupuncture

Depending on your location, there are a number of resources to expand your knowledge and exposure to these treatments. There are online resources such as www.yinyanghouse.com that offer additional information that ranges from historical background to individual point location for this type of therapy.

Also, if you would like to have acupuncture treatments at a teaching facility in your area, check these links to find a certified acupuncture school near you.

http://www.acupuncturetoday.com/schools/

http://www.acaom.org/find-a-school/

In addition, you can search individual states' professional licensing boards for qualified acupuncturists.

SMELL: Herbs, Flowers, Plants, and Essential Oils

There are countless online and retail sources for essential oils (EOs). The important thing is to use reputable sites and retailers for your product. A few general guidelines would be to use EOs that are 100% pure and natural not synthetic. Search for items that list the ingredients of the aromatherapy product as a specified plant species (e.g., *Lavandula officinalis* for Lavender EO). Other things to look for are the country of origin of the plant, how it was processed (e.g., distilled), and how it was grown (e.g., organic, wild-crafted, etc.).

Here are a few ideas to assist you in sourcing your EO:

- Local health food stores or grocery stores with natural health products (e.g., Whole Foods, Fresh Market)
- Online: There are many options. We list a few here in alphabetical order.
  - Aura Cacia: www.auracacia.com/essential-oil-directory.php
  - Floracopeia: www.floracopeia.com/
  - Mountain Rose Herbs: www.mountainroseherbs.com/catalog/aromatherapy
  - Organic Infusions: http://www.organicinfusionswholesale.com/essential-oils/

TASTE: Tea and Herbal Tisanes

As with EO options for aromatherapy oils, choices for sourcing your tea and herbals are large and varied. A few things to keep in mind when purchasing these products: look for the actual tea or herb name to be included in the ingredient list on the box/packaging. Avoid additives, artificial flavors and colors, as well as sugar.

The tea and herbs discussed in this book can be found in both loose leaf and individual teabag form. Many of the herbs—chamomile, ginger, and peppermint, to name just a few—are readily available on store shelves in the health food or tea sections. Some of the shops mentioned above for essential oil sourcing carry tea and herbal tisanes as well.

With tea drinking on the rise, there are also a number of tea shops, both chains and some wonderful individual tea purveyors that offer the items listed in our "TASTE" treatment protocol sections. Many of these same shops also offer online purchasing, and the tea can be shipped to your home. Here are a few examples of stores offering natural teas.

- Buddha Teas: www.buddhateas.com
- David's Tea: www.davidstea.com
- Mighty Leaf: www.mightyleaf.com
- Tealuxe: www.tealuxe.com
- Whole Foods: www.wholefoodsmarket.com/department/coffee-tea

SIGHT: Yoga Postures

There are a dizzying array of websites as well as yoga studios, centers, and retreat facilities to grow and augment your yoga practice. Here are just a few examples.

- Online, there are subscription services that offer all levels of yoga instruction videos, from $8–14 per month. www.gaia.com; www.oneoeight.tv; www.theyogacollective.com; www.grokker.com are a few comprehensive sites.
- Many local community centers, churches, and most YMCA's have yoga classes on their group fitness schedules. Find your nearest "Y" location at www.ymca.net.
- If you can steal away for a few days, a yoga retreat is a good way to jumpstart or reinforce your commitment to practice. There are hundreds of locations around the country, usually in quiet, beautiful places, ranging from the

high-end luxurious types to those that are simple and rustic. Here is one resource for budget-conscious clients: www.bookyogaretreats.com/all/c/budget-retreats/d/the-americas-and-caribbean/usa

SOUND: Sound and Music Therapy

Ask anyone, and they can likely name a few websites, apps, or other sources to download or stream music. Some are free and others charge a fee. Individual tastes and choices in music vary widely. Here are a few options, although the list is vast.

Music on Your Phone

In your iPhone's "App Store," search (using the magnifying glass icon) for example, "binaural beats." These are tone patterns based on beat frequency and contain no lyrics. There are several apps you can download for free or for a small charge. Choose an app that has the soundtracks categorized by moods and treatment goals, such as "promote sleep" or "increase alertness," or "relax."

To download popular songs on your iPhone, go to the iTunes Store icon, and search for individual songs you can download for a fee. Or, using the App Store icon, search for free streaming services such as "Spotify." Download that app for free, and you can search individual songs and artists for immediate playback. The only catch is you will be subjected to occasional advertisements. For a fee, you can upgrade your service to remove the ads. A free app called "Musi" will play music for you from anywhere on YouTube. The list goes on.

For Android phones, go to the "Play Store" icon and use the search bar at the top to find "Google Play Music," "Soundcloud," "Music Paradise," or "Spotify" just to name a few options. These apps will allow you to stream or download specific songs or artists either for free or for a small fee, and may or may not contain ads.

Sound Healing Tools

This may not be your first choice for sound therapy, but Tibetan Singing Bowls offer a rich and soothing variety of sounds that have been used by doctors to treat post-traumatic stress disorder. But their everyday value is to help bring the mind into awareness and create a relaxed, focused state. Here is a resource for Tibetan Singing Bowls: http://bestsingingbowls.com/sound-therapy/

Ohm Therapeutics is a popular manufacturer of tuning forks, the frequencies of which promote healing, relaxation, meditation, and pain management. Instructions are included. Ohm products can be purchased on Amazon, and information about their tuning forks can be found here: http://www.soundhealingtools.com/site.php?p=products&sp=tuning_forks

References

/////////////////////////////

ADHD in Teens. (2015). WebMD. Retrieved from http://www.webmd.com/add-adhd/childhood-adhd/adhd-teens

Agosti, R., Duke, R. K., Chrubasik, J. E., & Chrubasik, S. (2006). Effectiveness of *Petasites hybridus* preparations in the prophylaxis of migraine: A systematic review. *Phytomedicine,13*(9–10), 743–746.

Akhondzadeh, S., Kashani, L., Mobaseri, M., et al. (2001). Passionflower in the treatment of opiates withdrawal: a double-blind randomized controlled trial. *Journal of Clinical Pharmacy and Therapeutics*, 25:369–73.

Akhondzade, S., Tahmacebi-Pour, N., Noorbala, A. A., Amini, H., Fallah-Pour, H., Jamshidi, A. H., & Khani, M. (2005). Crocus sativus in the treatment of mild to moderate depression: A double-blind, randomized and placebo-controlled trial. *Phytotherapy Research, 19*, 148–151.

Altun A., & Ugur-Altun B. (2007). Melatonin: therapeutic and clinical utilization. *International Journal of Clinical Practice*. 61(5), 835–45.

American Academy of Child and Adolescent Psychology. (2001). The teen brain: Behavior, problem solving and decision making. Retrieved from https://www.aacap.org/AACAP/Families_and_Youth/Facts_for_Families/FFF-Guide/The-Teen-Brain-Behavior-Problem-Solving-and-Decision-Making-095.aspx

American Music Therapy Association. (2014). Music therapy and military populations: A status report and recommendations on music therapy treatment, programs, research, and practice policy. Retrieved from http://www.musictherapy.org/assets/1/7/MusicTherapyMilitaryPops_2014.pdf

American Psychological Association. (2015). Stress: The different kinds of stress. Retrieved from http://www.apa.org/helpcenter/stress-kinds.aspx.

American Psychiatric Association. (2013). Diagnostic and statistical manual of mental disorders (5th ed.). Washington, DC: Author.

Antrim, D. K. (1944). Music therapy. *Musical Quarterly, 30*, 409–420.

Anxiety and Depression Association of America. (2015). Complementary and alternative treatment. Retrieved from http://www.adaa.org/finding-help/treatment/complementary-alternative-treatment

Ardiel, E. L. (2010). The importance of touch in development. *Pediatric Child Health, 15*, 153–156.

Arnett, J. J. (2000). Emerging adulthood: A theory of development from the late teens through the twenties. *American Psychologist, 55*, 469–480.

Avallone, R., Zanoli, P., Corsi, L., Cannazza, G., Baraldi, M. (1996). Benzodiazepine compounds and GABA in flower heads of matricaria chamomilla. *Phytotherapy Research*, 10:177–179.

Awad, R., Levac, D., Cybulska, P., Merali, Z., Trudeau, V.L., Arnason JT (2007). Effects of traditionally used anxiolytic botanicals on enzymes of the gamma-aminobutyric acid (GABA) system. *Canadian Journal of Physiology and Pharmacology, 85*(9):933–42.

Balentine, D., Wiserman, S. A., & Bouwens, L. C. M. (1997). The chemistry of tea flavonoids. *Critical Reviews in Food Science and Nutrition, 37*, 693–704.

Banks, S., & Dinges, D. (2007). Behavioral and physiological consequences of sleep restriction. *Journal of Clinical Sleep Medicine, 3*, 519–528.

Beckhuis, T. (2009). Music therapy may reduce pain and anxiety in children undergoing medical and dental procedures. *Journal of Evidence-Based Dental Practice, 9*, 213–214.

Beddoe, A. E., Paul Yang, C. P., Kennedy, H. P., Weiss, S. J., & Lee, K. A. (2009). The effects of mindfulness-based yoga during pregnancy on maternal psychological and physical distress. *Journal of Obstetric Gynecologic and Neonatal Nursing, 38*, 310–319.

Beithon, J., et al. (2013). Diagnosis and treatment of headache. Bloomington, MN: Institute for Clinical Systems Improvement.

Big Toe Pose. (2015, August 21). *Yoga Journal.* Retrieved from http://www
.yogajournal.com/pose/big-toe-pose/

Biranholz, J., & Benacerraf, B. (1983). The development of human fetal hearing.
Science (New Series), *222,* 516–518.

Blackwell, D., & Clarke, T. C. (2013). QuickStats: Percentage of adults who often
felt very tired or exhausted in the past 3 months, by sex and age group—
National Health Interview Survey, United States, 2010–2011. *MMWR, 62*(14),
275. Retrieved from http://www.cdc.gov/mmwr/preview/mmwrhtml/
mm6214a5.htm

Blau, J. N. (1992). Migraine: Theories of pathogenesis. *Lancet, 339,* 1202–1207.

Blumenthal, J. A., Babyak, M. A., Doraiswamy, P. M., Watkins, L., Hoffman, B. M.,
Barbour, K. A., et al. (2007). Exercise and pharmacotherapy in the treatment
of major depressive disorder. *Psychosomatic Medicine, 69,* 587–596.

Boksem, M. A. S., & Tops, M. (2008). Mental fatigue: Costs and benefits. *Brain
Research Reviews, 59,* 125–139.

Bowen, S., Witkiewitz, K., Clifasefi, S. L., Grow, J., Chawla, N., Hsu, S. H., et al.
(2014). Relative efficacy of mindfulness-based relapse prevention, standard
relapse prevention, and treatment as usual for substance use disorders: A
randomized clinical trial. *JAMA Psychiatry, 71,* 547–556.

Bradt, J., Dileo, C., & Potvin, N. (2009). Music for stress and anxiety reduction in coronary heart disease patients. *Cochrane Database of Systematic
Reviews, 4,* Art. No. CD006566. Retrieved from http://onlinelibrary.wiley.
com/doi/10.1002/14651858.CD006577.pub3/full

Brand, S., Gerber, M., Beck, J., Hatzinger, M., Pühse, U., & Holsboer-Trachsler, E.
(2010). High exercise levels are related to favorable sleep patterns and psychological functioning in adolescents: A comparison of athletes and controls.
Journal of Adolescent Health, 46, 133–141.

Breslin, K. T., Reed, M. R., & Malone, S. B. (2003). An holistic approach to substance abuse treatment. *Journal of Psychoactive Drugs, 35,* 247–251.

Brody, G. E., Beach, S. R., Philibert, R. A., Chen, Y. F., & Murry, V. M. (2009).
Prevention effects moderate the association of 5-HTTLPR and youth risk
behavior initiation: Gene × environment hypotheses tested via a randomized
prevention design. *Child Development, 80,* 645–661.

Brown, K. W., Ryan, R. M., & Creswell, J. D. (2007). Mindfulness: Theoretical
foundations and evidence for its salutary effects. *Psychological Inquiry:*

An International Journal for the Advancement of Psychological Theory, 18, 211–237.

Brown, R. P., & Gerbarg, P. L. (2012). *Non-drug treatments for ADHD: New options for kids, adults, and clinicians.* New York, NY: W. W. Norton & Company.

Burns, D. (2001). The effect of the Bonny method of guided imagery and music on the mood and life quality of cancer patients. *Journal of Music Therapy, 38,* 51–65.

Calabro, S. (2012). "Why are you doing that point?" Liver 3 and Large Intestine 4. AcuTake, February 7. Retrieved from http://acutakehealth.com/why-are-you-doing-that-point-lv3-li4

Cai, Na, et al. (2015). Sparse whole-genome sequencing identifies two loci for major depressive disorder. *Nature, 523,* 588–591.

Campbell, P. S., Connell, C., & Beegle, A. (2007). Adolescents' expressed meanings of music in and out of school. *Journal of Research in Music Education, 55,* 220–236.

Cases, J. (2010). Leaf extract in the treatment of volunteers suffering from mild-to-moderate anxiety disorders and sleep disturbances. *Mediterranean Journal of Nutrition and Metabolism, 4,* 211–218.

Cerny, A., Shmid, K. (1999) Tolerability and efficacy of valerian/lemon balm in healthy volunteers (a double blind, placebo-controlled, multicentre study). *Fitoterapia,* 70:221–8.

Chollot, R. (2013, March 11). The power of touch. *Psychology Today.* Retrieved from https://www.psychologytoday.com/articles/201302/the-power-touch

Chudler, E. H. (2015, March). Brain facts and figures. Retrieved from https://faculty.washington.edu/chudler/facts.html.

Cieza, A., Maier, P., & Poppel, E. (2003). Effects of Ginkgo biloba on mental functioning in healthy volunteers. *Archives of Medical Research* 34(5):373–381.

Cohen, S., & Janicki-Deverts, D. (2012). Who's stressed? Distributions of psychological stress in the United States in probability samples from 1983, 2006, and 2009. *Journal of Applied Psychology, 42,* 1320–1334.

Colquhoun, D., & Novella, S. P. (2013, June). Acupuncture is theatrical placebo. *Anesthesia and Analgesia, 116,* 1360–1363.

Colten H. R., & Altevogt B. M. (Eds.). (2006). Sleep disorders and sleep deprivation: an unmet public health problem. Washington, DC: National Academies Press (US). Available from: http://www.ncbi.nlm.nih.gov/books/NBK19960/

Cook, P. M. (1997). Sacred music therapy in North India. *World of Music, 39*, 61–83.

Cruse, R. P. (2015). Pathophysiology, clinical features, and diagnosis of migraine in children. UpToDate. Retrieved from http://www.uptodate.com/contents/pathophysiology-clinical-features-and-diagnosis-of-migraine-in-children

Curcio, G., Ferrara, M., & De Gennaro, L. (2006). Sleep loss, learning capacity and academic performance. *Sleep Medicine Reviews, 10*, 323–337.

Cuvellier, J. C. (2009). Management of chronic daily headache in children and adolescents. *Revue Neurologique, 165*, 521–531.

Dalla Libera, D., Colombo, B., Pavan, G., & Comi, G. (2014). Complementary and alternative medicine (CAM) use in an Italian cohort of pediatric headache patients: The tip of the iceberg. *Neurological Sciences, 35*, 145.

Davis, M., Matthews, K. A., & Twamley, E. W. (1990). Is life more difficult on Mars or Venus? A meta-analytic review of sex differences in major and minor life events. *Annals of Behavioral Medicine, 21*, 83–97.

Deka, A., & Vita, J. A. (2011). Tea and cardiovascular disease. *Pharmacological Research, 64*(2), 136–145. doi:10.1016/j.phrs.2011.03.009

Devol, R., & Bedroussian, A. (2007). An unhealthy America: The economic burden of chronic disease. Milken Institute. Retrieved from http://assets1c.milkeninstitute.org/assets/Publication/ResearchReport/PDF/chronic_disease_report.pdf

Dhond, R. P., Kettner, N., & Napadow, V. (2007). Neuroimaging acupuncture effects in the human brain. *Journal of Alternative and Complementary Medicine, 13*, 603–616.

Diener, H. C., Pfaffenrath, V., Schnitker, J., Friede, M., & Henneicke-von Zepelin, H. H. (2005). Efficacy and safety of 6.25 mg t.i.d. feverfew CO2-extract (MIG-99) in migraine prevention—a randomized, double-blind, multicentre, placebo-controlled study. *Cephalalgia, 25*, 1031–1041.

Dixit, S., Agrawal, U., & Dubey, G. (1993). Executive fatigue and its management with Mentat. *Pharmacopsychoecologia, 6*, 7–9, 20–25.

Dryden-Edwards, R. (2015). Teen drug abuse. Medicine.net. Retrieved from http://www.medicinenet.com/script/main/art.asp?articlekey=81937

Dusek, J. A., et al. (2008). Stress management versus lifestyle modification on systolic hypertension and medication elimination: A randomized trial. *Journal of Alternative and Complementary Medicine, 14*, 129–138.

Edwards, J. (2007). *Music: Promoting health and creating community in health-care contexts.* Newcastle, UK: Cambridge Scholars.

EFSA Panel on Dietetic Products, Nutrition and Allergies (2012). Scientific opinion on the suitability of goat milk protein as a source of protein in infant formulae and in follow-on formulae. *EFSA Journal*, 10(3), 2603.

Ekkekakis, P., Hargreaves, E. A., & Parfitt, E. A. (2013). Invited guest editorial: Envisioning the next fifty years of research on the exercise-affect relationship. *Physiology of Sport and Exercise, 14*, 751–758.

Epel, E. S., & Lithgow, G. J. (2014). Stress biology and aging mechanisms: Toward understanding the deep connection between adaptation to stress longevity. *Journal of Gerontology, Biological Sciences and Medical Sciences, 69*(Suppl. 1), 10–16.

Errington-Evans, N. (2011). Acupuncture for anxiety. *CNS Neurosciences and Therapeutics, 18*, 277–284.

Eshkevari, L., Permaul, E., & Mulroney, E. (2003). Acupuncture blocks cold stress-induced increases in the hypothalamus-pituitary-adrenal axis in the rat. *Journal of Endocrinology, 217*, 995–1104.

European Medicines Agency (EMA) Committee on Herbal Medicinal Products. (2011). Final community herbal monograph on *Cinnamomum verum* J.S. Presl, cortex. London, UK: *EMA*. Retrieved May 10, 2011 from www.ema.europa .eu/docs/en_GB/document_library/Herbal_-_Community_herbal_ monograph/2011/08/WC500110095.pdf.

Evans, W., & Lambert, C. P. (2007). Physiological basis of fatigue. *American Journal of Physical Medicine and Rehabilitation, 86*, S29–S46.

Field, T. (2002). Infants' need for touch. *Human Development, 45*, 100–103.

Field, Martinez, Nawrocki, Pickens, Fox, & Schanberg. (1998). Music shifts frontal EEG in depressed adolescents. *Adolescence*, 33 (129), 109–116.

Findlay, S. M. (2008). The tired teen: A review of the assessment and management of the adolescent with sleepiness and fatigue. *Pediatrics and Child Health, 13*, 37–42.

Fisher, M. (2003). Fatigue in adolescents. *Journal of Pediatric and Adolescent Gynecology, 26*, 252–256.

Flexer, C. (2011, July 25). The auditory brain: Conversations for pediatric audiologists. Audiology Online. Retrieved from http://www.audiologyonline.com/ articles/auditory-brain-conversations-for-pediatric-817

Freedman, P. (2007). *Food: The history of taste.* California Studies in Food and Culture, Vol. 21. Oakland: University of California Press.

Fukada, K., Straus, S. E., Hickie, I., Sharpe, M. C., Dobbins, J. G., & Komaroff, A. (1994). The chronic fatigue syndrome: A comprehensive approach to its definition and study. *Annals of Internal Medicine, 121,* 953–959.

Gaylord, S. A., & Mann, D. (2007). Rationales for CAM education in health professions training programs. *Academic Medicine, 82,* 927–933.

Gaynor, M. (2002). *The healing power of sound: Recovery from life-threatening illness using sound, voice, and music* (Boston: Shambhala.

Geleijnse, J. M., Launer, L. J., Van der Kuip, D. A., Hofman, A., & Witteman, J. C. (2002). Inverse association of tea and flavonoid intakes with incident myocardial infarction: The Rotterdam Study. *American Journal of Clinicial Nutrition, 75*(5), 880–886.

Goldman, L. S., Genel, M., Bezman, R. J., & Slanetz, P. J. (1998). Diagnosis and treatment of attention-deficit hyperactivity disorder in children and adolescents. *JAMA, 279,* 1100–1107.

Goleman, D. (2013). *Focus: The hidden driver of excellence.* New York: Harper.

Grady, D. (1993, June). The vision thing: Mainly in the brain. *Discover.* Retrieved from http://discovermagazine.com/1993/jun/thevisionthingma227

Greenlaw, E. (2010). Getting right: Eating right for depression. WebMD. Retrieved from http://www.webmd.com/depression/features/diet-for-depression?print=true

Guidetti, V., & Galli, F. (2008). Evolution of headache in childhood and adolescence: An 8-year follow-up. *Cephalalgia, 18,* 449–454.

Hagen, S. (2012). The mind's eye. *Rochester Review, 74*(4), 32–37.

Hahn, E. J., Rayens, M. K., Chaloupka, F. J., Okoli, C. T. C., & Yang, J. (2002). Projected smoking-related deaths among U.S. youth: A 2000 update. ImpacTeen Research Paper Series, No. 22. Retrieved from http://www.impacteen.org/generalarea_PDFs/Hahn_researchpaper22_May2002.pdf

Halverson, J. H., et al. (2015) Depression. *Medscape: Drugs and Disease,* Retrieved from http://emedicine.medscape.com/article/286759-overview.

Hanley, J., Stirling, P., & Brown, C. (2003). Randomised controlled trial of therapeutic massage in the management of stress. *British Journal of General Practice, 53,* 486.

Harding, A., & Clark, L. (2014). Pediatric migraine: Common, yet treatable. *Nurse Practitioner, 39*, 22–31.

Harris, M. J. (2014). Music as a transition for sleep. *Occupational Therapy Now, 16*(6), 11–13.

Hershey, A. D., Kabbouche, M. A., & Powers, S. W. (2006). Chronic daily headaches in children. *Current Pain and Headache Reports, 10*, 370–376.

Herz, R. S. (2009). Aromatherapy facts and fictions: A scientific analysis of olfactory effects on mood, psychology and behavior. *International Journal of Neuroscience, 119*, 263–290.

Hobson, J. A. (2009). REM sleep and dreaming: Towards a theory of consciousness. *Nature Reviews Neuroscience, 10*, 803–813.

Hoffman, D. L., Dukes, E. M., & Wittchen, H. -U. (2008). Human and economic burden of generalized anxiety disorder. *Depression and Anxiety*, 25, 72–90.

Hohl, J. V., Atzmueller, M., Fink, B., & Grammer, K. (2001). Human pheromones: Integrating neuroendocrinology and ethology. *Neuroendocrinology Letters, 22*, 309–321.

Holt-Lunstad, J., Smith, T. B., & Layton, J. B. (2010). Social relationships and mortality risk: A meta-analytic review. *PLOS Medicine, 7*, e1000316.

Hong, J. -W., et al. (2012). Anti-inflammatory activity of cinnamon water extract in vivo and in vitro LPS-induced models. *BMC Central Complementary and Alternative Medicine,* The official journal of the International Society for Complementary Medicine Research (ISCMR), 12.1: 237.

Hou, W. H., Chiang, P. T., Hsu, T. Y., Chiu, S. Y., & Yen, Y. C. (2010). Treatment effects of massage therapy in depressed people: A meta-analysis. *Journal of Clinical Psychiatry, 71*, 894–301.

Hoyert, D. L., & Xu, J. (2012). Deaths: Final data from 2011. *National Vital Statistics Reports, 61*(6).

Ishak, W. (2011). The impact of psychotherapy, pharmacotherapy, and their combination on quality of life in depression. *Harvard Review of Psychiatry, 19*, 277–289.

James, W. (1987). Letter to *Boston Evening Transcript* (March 17, 1894). In W.James, *Essays, comments, and reviews.* Cambridge, MA: Harvard University Press.

Jang, J., et al. (2011) Suppression of growth and invasive behavior of human prostate cancer cells by ProstaCaidTM: Mechanism of activity. *International*

Journal of Oncology. 38(6): 1675–82. http://www.spandidos-publications. com/ijo/38/6/1675.

Jensen, F. E., & Nutt, A. E. (2015). *The teenage brain: A neuroscientist's survival guide to raising adolescents and young adults.* New York: Harper.

Jindal, V., Ge, A., & Mansky, P. J. (2008). Safety and efficacy of acupuncture in children: A review of the evidence. *Journal of Pediatric/Oncology, 30,* 431–442.

Johannes, J. (2010). A scent to lull you to sleep. *Wall Street Journal,* August 24. Retrieved from http://www.wsj.com/articles/SB10001424052748703846604 5755447591695802182

Johnston, L. D., et al. (2008). *Monitoring the future: National results on adolescent drug abuse: Overview of key findings.* Bethesda, MD: National Institute of Drug Abuse, National Institute of Health, U.S. Department of Health and Human Services.

Kabat-Zinn, J. (1990). *Full catastrophe living.* New York: Bantam Dell.

Kabbouche, M. A., & Gilman, D. K. (2008). Management of migraine in adolescents. *Journal of Neuropsychiatric Disease and Treatment, 4,* 535–548.

Kalivas, P. W., & Volkow, N. D. (2005). The neural basis of addiction: A pathology of motivation and choice. *American Journal of Psychiatry, 162,* 1403–1413.

Kaplan, G. (1997). A brief history of acupuncture's journey to the West. *Journal of Alternative and Complementary Medicine, 3,* S5–S10.

Keller, M. C., & Nesse, R. (2005). Is low mood an adaptation? Evidence for subtypes with symptoms that match precipitants. *Journal of Affective Disorders, 86,* 27–35.

Kessler, R. C., & Greenberg, P. E. (2002). The economic burden of anxiety and stress disorders. *Neuropsychopharmacology: The fifth generation of progress, 67,* 982–992.

Kiecolt-Glaser, J. K., Graham, J. E., Malarkey, W. B., Porter, K., Lemeshow, S., & Glaser, R. (2008). Olfactory influences on mood and autonomic, endocrine, and immune function. *Psychoneuroendocrinology, 33*(3), 328–339.

Kim, J. T., Wajda, M., Cuff, G., Serota, D., Schlame, M., Axelrod, D. M., Guth, A. A., & Bekker, A. Y. (2006). Evaluation of aromatherapy in treating postoperative pain: Pilot study. *Pain Practice, 6*(4), 273–277.

Ko, S.-J. (2012). Effect of oriental medicine music therapy on idiopathic chronic fatigue. *European Journal of Integrative Medicine, 4,* e41–e44.

Koch, S. C., Morlinghaus, K., & Fuch, T. (2007). The joy dance: Specific effects of a single dance intervention on psychiatric patients with depression. *Arts in Psychotherapy, 34*, 340–349.

Komori T, et al. (1995). Application of fragrances to treatments for depression. *Japanese Journal of Psychopharmacology*, 15(1):39–42.

Koob, G., & Kreek, M. J. (2007). Stress, dysregulation of drug reward pathways, and the transition to drug dependence. *America Journal of Psychiatry, 164*, 1149–1159.

Kringelbach, M. (2004). Food for thought: Hedonic experience beyond homeostasis in the human brain. *Neuroscience, 126*, 807–819.

Krueger, J. M., Rector, D. M., Roy, S., Van Dongen, H. P. A., Belenky, G., & Panksepp, J. (2008). Sleep as a fundamental property of neuronal assemblies. *Nature Reviews Neuroscience, 9*, 910–919.

Kuriyama, H. (2005). Immunological and psychological benefits of aromatherapy massage. *Evidence-Based Complementary and Alternative Medicine, 2*, 179–184.

Lasky, R. E., & Klein, R. E. (1979). The reaction of five-month-old infants to eye contact of the mother and of a stranger. *Merrill-Palmer Quarterly of Behavior and Development, 25*, 163–170.

Lavender. (2015). University of Maryland Medical Center. Retrieved from http://umm.edu/health/medical/altmed/herb/lavender

Law, D., Baxter, G. D., & Tumilty, S. (2015). Acupuncture for treating musculoskeletal pain: A systematic review with meta-analysis. *Journal of Acupuncture Meridian Studies*, 8(1), 2e16.

Levine, D. A. (2007). "Pharming": The abuse of prescription and over-the-counter drugs in teens. *Current Opinion in Pediatrics, 19*, 270–274.

Lian, M., Moruraux, A., & Iannetti, G. (2011). Parallel processing of nociceptive and non-nociceptive somatosensory information in the human primary and secondary somatosensory cortices: Evidence from dynamic causal modeling of functional magnetic resonance imaging data. *Journal of Neuroscience, 31*, 8976–8985.

Liem, D. G., & Mennella, J. A. (2003). Heightened sour preferences during childhood. *Chemical Senses, 28*, 173–180.

Lim, H. A., Miller, K., & Fabian, C. (2011). The effects of therapeutic instrumental music performance on endurance level, self-perceived fatigue level, and self-perceived exertion of inpatients in physical rehabilitation. *Journal of Music Therapy, 48*, 124–148.

Lin, Y. (1995). Acupuncture treatment for insomnia and acupuncture analgesia. *Psychiatry and Clinical Neurosciences*, 49: 119–120. doi: 10.1111/j.1440-1819.1995.tb01874.x

Lind, B. K., Lafferty, W. E., Tyree, P. T., & Diehr, P. K. (2010). Comparison of health care expenditures among insured users and nonusers of complementary and alternative medicine in Washington State: A cost minimization analysis. *Journal of Alternative and Complementary Medicine, 16*(4), 411–417.

Ljubinovic, N. (2015, May). Acupuncture, anxiety and depression. Psych Central. Retrieved from http://psychcentral.com/lib/acupuncture-anxiety-depression/

Lo, M. Y., Lin, J.-G., Ong, M. W., & Sun, W.-Z. (2013). Cerebral hemodynamic responses to acupuncture in migraine patients: A systematic review. *Journal of Traditional Complementary Medicine, 3*, 213–220.

Lu, S., Fuh, J., Wang, S., Juang, K.-D., Chen, S.-P., Liao, Y.-C., & Wang, Y.-F. (2013). Incidence and risk factors of chronic daily headache in young adolescents: A school cohort study. *Pediatrics, 132*, 9–16.

Lu, K., Gray, M. A., Oliver, C., Liley, D. T., Harrison, B. J., Bartholomeusz, C. F., Phan, K. L., & Nathan, P. J. (2004). The acute effects of L-theanine in comparison with alprazolam on anticipatory anxiety in humans. *Human Psychopharmacology, 29*, 457–465.

Mack, K. J. (2009). New daily persistent headache in children and adults. *Current Pain and Headache Reports, 13,* 47–51.

Magistrelli A., & Chezem J. C. (2012). Effect of ground cinnamon on postprandial blood glucose concentration in normal-weight and obese adults. *Journal of the Academy of Nutrition and Dietetics.* 2012 Nov;112(11):1806–9. doi: 10.1016/j.jand.2012.07.037.

Maizes, V., Rakel, D., & Niemiec, C. (2009). Integrative medicine and patient-centered care. *Explore, 5,* 277–289.

Mandel, S. A., Amit, T., Kalfon, L., Reznichenko, L., & Youdim, M. B. H. (2008). Targeting multiple neurodegenerative disease etiologies with multimodal-acting green tea catechins. *Journal of Nutrition,138*, 1578S–1583S.

Maratos, A., Crawford, M. J., & Procter, S. (2011). Music therapy for depression: It seems to work, but how? *British Journal of Psychiatry, 199*, 92–93.

Martyn-Nemeth, P., Penckofer, S., Gulanick, M., Velsor-Friedrich, B., & Bryant, F. B.

(2009). The relationships among self-esteem, stress, coping, eating behavior, and depressive mood in adolescents. *Research in Nursing and Health, 32,* 96–109.

May, A., Ashburner, J., Büchel, C., McGonigle, D. J., Friston, K. J., Frackowiak, R. S. J., & Goadsby, P. J. (1999). Correlation between structural and functional changes in brain in an idiopathic headache syndrome. *Nature Medicine, 5,* 836–838.

Mayo Clinic. (2013a, March 5). Attention-deficit/hyperactivity disorder (ADHD) in children. Retrieved from http://www.mayoclinic.org/diseases-conditions/ adhd/basics/definition/con-20023647

Mayo Clinic. (2013b). Diseases and conditions: Cluster headache: Definition. Retrieved from http://www.mayoclinic.org/diseases-conditions/ cluster-headache/basics/definition/con-20031706

Mayo Clinic. (2013c). Diseases and conditions: Migraine: Definition. Retrieved from http://www.mayoclinic.org/diseases-conditions/migraine-headache/ basics/definition/con-20026358

Mayo Clinic. (2013d). Diseases and conditions: Tension headache: Definition. Retrieved from http://www.mayoclinic.org/diseases-conditions/ tension-headache/basics/definition/con-20014295

Mayo Clinic. (2013e, June 4). Symptoms: Headache: Causes. Retrieved from http:// www.mayoclinic.org/symptoms/headache/basics/causes/sym-20050800

McCall, T. (2007). *Yoga as medicine.* New York: Bantam.

McEwen, B. S. (2002). Protective and damaging effects of stress mediators: The good and bad sides of the response to stress. *Metabolism Clinical Experimental, 51*(Suppl. 1), 2–4.

McEwen, B. S. (2004). Protection and damage from acute and chronic stress: Allostasis and allostatic overload and relevance to the pathophysiology of psychiatric disorders. *Annals of the New York Academy of Sciences, 1032,* 1–7.

McFadden, K., Healy, K. M., Dettman, M. L., Kaye, J. T., Ito, T. A., & Hernández, T. D. (2011). Acupressure as a non-pharmacological intervention for traumatic brain injury (TBI). *Journal of Neurotrauma, 28*(1), 21–34.

Medical News Today. (2015, September) What is tiredness or fatigue? How can I beat tiredness? Retrieved from http://www.medicalnewstoday.com/ articles/8877.php#what_is_fatigue

Menghini, L.,et al. (2010) Antiproliferative, protective and antioxidant effects of artichoke, dandelion, tumeric, and rosemary extracts and their formulation. *International Journal of Immunopathology and Pharmacology*, 23(2): 601–10. http://www.ncbi.nlm.nih.gov/pubmed/20646355.

Miller, L. H., Smith, A. D. & Rothstein, L. (1994) *The Stress Solution: An Action Plan to Manage the Stress in Your Life*. Pocket Books, p. 24.

Miller, N. S., & Giannini, A. J. (1990). The disease model of addiction. *Journal of Psychoactive Drugs, 22*, 83–85.

Mindell, J., Owens, J., & Carskadon, M. A. (1999). Developmental features of sleep. *Child and Adolescent Psychiattric Clinics of North America, 4*, 695–725.

Misic, P., Arandjelovic, D., Stanojkovic, S., Vladejic, S., & Mladenovic, J. (2010). Music therapy. *European Psychiatry, 25*(Suppl. 1), 839.

Miyasaka, L. S., Atallah, A. N., Soares, B. G. (2007). Passiflora for anxiety disorder. *Cochrane Database of Systematic Reviews*, (1):CD004518.

Montagu, A. (1984). The skin, touch and human development. *Clinics in Dermatology, 2*, 17–26.

Moore, J., & Linthicum, F., Jr. (2007). The human auditory system: A timeline of development. *International Journal of Audiology, 46*, 460–478.

Moreland, C. S., & Bonin, L. (2015). Information: Depression treatment options for adolescents (beyond the basics). UpToDate. Retrieved from http://www.uptodate.com/contents/depression-treatment-options-for-children-and-adolescents-beyond-the-basics

Morgan, S., Littman, L., Palmer, C., Singh, G., & LaRiccia, P. J. (2012). A short guide to peer-reviewed, MEDLINE-indexed complementary and alternative medicine journals. *Holistic Nursing Practice, 26*(3), 164–172. doi: 10.1097/HNP.0b013e31824ef4fd

Moturi, S., & Avis, K. (2010). Assessment and treatment of common pediatric sleep disorders. *Psychiatry, 7*, 24–37.

Moyer, C. A., Rounds, J., & Hannum, J. W. (2004). A meta-analysis of massage therapy research. *Psychological Bulletin, 130*, 3–18.

Murray, C. J. L., & Lopez, A. D. (Eds.). (1996). *The global burden of disease: A comprehensive assessment of mortality and disability from diseases, injuries and risk factors in 1990 and projected to 2020.* Cambridge, MA: Harvard School of Public Health.

National Center for Complementary and Integrative Health. (2013, June). Yoga for health. Retrieved from https://nccih.nih.gov/health/yoga/introduction.htm

National Geographic Channel. (2011, September 16). Facts about perception. Retrieved from http://channel.nationalgeographic.com/channel/brain-games/articles/brain-games-watch-this-perception-facts/.

National Geographic TV. (2015, August 3). Brain games: You won't believe your eyes. Retrieved from http://natgeotv.com.au/tv/brain-games/brain-games-you-wont-believe-your-eyes.aspx

National Institute of Mental Health. (2015a, May). Anxiety disorders. Retrieved from http://www.nimh.nih.gov/health/topics/anxiety-disorders/index.shtml

National Institute of Mental Health. (2015b). Depression in children and adolescents. Retrieved from http://www.nimh.nih.gov/health/topics/depression-in-children-and-adolescents/index.shtml

National Institute of Mental Health. (2015c). Major depression among adolescents. Retrieved from http://www.nimh.nih.gov/health/statistics/prevalence/major-depression-among-adolescents.shtml

National Institute of Mental Health. (2015d). Attention deficit hyperactivity disorder. Retrieved from http://www.nimh.nih.gov/health/publications/attention-deficit-hyperactivity-disorder-easy-to-read/index.shtml

National Institute on Drug Abuse. (2014). What are the long-term effects of heroin use? Retrieved from http://www.drugabuse.gov/publications/research-reports/heroin/what-are-long-term-effects-heroin-use

Nelson, R., Sur, M., & Kaas, J. H. (1980). Representations of the body surface in postcentral parietal cortex of *Macaca fascicularis*. *Journal of Comparative Neurology, 192*, 611–643.

Nettle, D. (2008). An evolutionary model of low mood states. *Journal of Theoretical Biology, 257*, 100–103.

Nobre, A. C., Rao, A., & Owen, G. N. (2008). L-theanine, a natural constituent in tea, and its effect on mental state. *Asia Pacific Journal of Clinical Nutrition, 17*(Suppl. 1), 167–168.

Nordqvist, J. (2015). Brain freeze: What is it? *Medical News Today*. Retrieved from http://www.medicalnewstoday.com/articles/244458.php

Oberhelman, S. M. (2013). Introduction: Medical pluralism, healing, and dreams in Greek culture. In S. M. Oberhelman (Ed.), *Dreams, healing, and medicine in Greece: From antiquity to the present* (1–33). Burlington, VT: Ashgate.

Oelkers-Ax, R., Leins, A., Parzer, P., Hillecke, T., Bolay, H. V., Fischer, J., Bender, S., Hermanns, U., & Resch, F. (2008). Butterbur root extract and music therapy in the prevention of childhood migraine: An explorative study. *European Journal of Pain, 12*, 301–313.

Pardo-Aldave, K., Diaz-Pizan, M. E., Villegas, L. F., et al. (2009). Child behavior modulation during first dental visit after administration of lemon balm. *International Journal of Pediatric Dentistry, 19*, 66–170.

Park, C. L., Armell, S., & Tennen, H. (2004). The daily stress and coping process and alcohol use among college students. *Journal of Studies on Alcohol, 65*, 126–135.

Parker-Hope, T. (2008). Using music to lift depression's veil. *New York Times*, January 24.

Pearson, N., & Chesney, M. (2007). The CAM education program of the National Center for Complementary and Alternative Medicine: An overview. *Academic Medicine, 82*, 921–926.

Pelletier, C. L. (2004). The effect of music on decreasing arousal due to stress: A meta-analysis. *Journal of Music Therapy, 41*, 192–214.

Perry, N., & Perry, E. (2006). Aromatherapy in the management of psychiatric disorders: Clinical and neuropharmacological perspectives. *CNS Drugs, 20*, 257–280.

Peters, U., Poole, C., & Arab, L. (2001). Does tea affect cardiovascular disease? A meta-analysis. *American Journal of Epidemiology, 154*(6), 495–503.

Pfaffenrath, V., Diener, H. C., Fischer, M., Friede, M., & Henneicke-von Zepelin, H. H. (2002). The efficacy and safety of Tanacetum parthenium (feverfew) in migraine prophylaxis—a double-blind, multicentre, randomized placebo-controlled dose-response study. *Cephalalgia, 22*, 523–532.

Pillai, A.K., Sharma, K.K., Gupta, Y.K., Bakhshi, S. (2011). Anti-emetic effect of ginger powder versus placebo as an add-on therapy in children and young adults receiving high emetogenic chemotherapy. *Pediatric Blood & Cancer*, 56(2):234–238.

Porter, S., Holmes, V., McLaughlin, K., Lynn, F., Cardwell, C., Braiden, H.-J., Doran, J., & Rogan, S. (2012). Music in mind: A randomized controlled trial of music therapy for young people with behavioural and emotional problems: Study protocol. *Journal of Advanced Nursing, 68*, 2349–2358. doi: 10.1111/j.1365-2648.2011.05936.x

Pothmann, R., & Danesch, U. (2005). Migraine prevention in children and adolescents: Results of an open study with a special butterbur root extract. *Headache, 45*, 196–203.

Rašković, A. ,Pavlovic, N., et al. (2015) Effects of pharmaceutical formulations containing thyme on carbon tetrachloride-induced liver injury in rats. *BMC Complementary and Alternative Medicine.* The Official Journal of the International Society for Complementary Medicine Research (ISCMR), 15:442.

Rea, S. (2007a, August 28). Bend back into your body: Cobra. *Yoga Journal.* Retrieved from http://www.yogajournal.com/article/beginners/bhujangasana-2/

Rea, S. (2007b, August 28). Find full-body joy in Downward-Facing Dog pose. *Yoga Journal.* Retrieved from http://www.yogajournal.com/article/beginners/adho-mukha-svanasana/

Reston, J. (1971, July 2). Now, about my operation in Peking. *New York Times.*

Rezai-Zadeh, K., Shytle, D., Sun, N., Mori, T., Hou, H., Jeanniton, D., Ehrhart, J., Townsend, K., Zeng, J., Morgan, D., Hardy, J., Town, T., & Tan, J. (2005). Green tea epigallocatechin-3-gallate (EGCG) modulates amyloid precursor protein cleavage and reduces cerebral amyloidosis in Alzheimer transgenic mice. *Journal of Neuroscience, 25*(38), 8807–8814.

Rice, F., Harold, G., & Thapar, A. (2002). The genetic aetiology of childhood depression: A review. *Journal of Child Psychology and Psychiatry, 43*, 65–79.

Richardson, K. M., & Rothstein, H. R. (2008). Effects of occupational stress management intervention programs: A meta-analysis. *Journal of Occupational Health Psychology, 13*(1), 69.

Roberts, J. (2013). Low mood and depression in adolescence. *British Journal of General Practice, 63*, 273–274.

Robson, K. S. (1967). The role of eye-to-eye contact in maternal-infant attachment. *Journal of Child Psychology and Psychiatry, 8*, 13–25.

Rodgers, A. L. (2012, Summer). Music: Sound medicine for ADHD. *ADDitude.* Retrieved from http://www.additudemag.com/adhd/article/9558-2.html

Roth, E. & Goldman, R. (2015). Understanding ADHD inattentive type. Healthline.com. Retrieved from http://www.healthline.com/health/adhd/inattentive-type#Overview1

Sadeh A., Gruber R., & Raviv A. (2003). The effects of sleep restriction and extension on school-age children: What a difference an hour makes. *Child Development*, 74 (2), 444–455.

Salehi B., Imani R., Mohammadi M.R., et al. (2010). Ginkgo bilboa for attention-deficit/hyperactivity disorder in children and adolescents: A double blind, randomized controlled trial. *Progress in Neuro-Psychopharmacology and Biological Psychiatry*, 34:76–80.

Samaha, E., Lal, S., Samaha, N., & Wyndham, J. (2007). Psychological, lifestyle and coping contributors to chronic fatigue in shift-worker nurses. *Journal of Advanced Nursing, 59*, 221–232.

Santos, E. L., Dias, B. H. M., de Andrade, A. C. R., Pascoal, A. M. H., Filho, F. E. V., Medeiros, F. C., & Guimarães, S. B. (2013). Effects of acupuncture and electroacupuncture on estradiol-induced inflammation and oxidative stress in healthy rodents. *Acta Cirugica Brasileira, 28*, 582–586.

Sasannejad, P., Saeedi, M., Shoeibi, A., Gorji, A., Abbasi, M., & Foroughipour, M. (2010). Lavender essential oil in the treatment of migraine headache: A placebo-controlled clinical trial. *European Neurology, 67*, 288–291.

Savic, I. (2002). Brain imaging studies of the functional organization of human olfaction. *Neuroscientist, 8*, 204–211.

Sawi, A., & Breuner, C. C. (2012). Complementary, holistic, and integrative medicine: Depression, sleep disorders, and substance abuse. *Pediatric Review, 33*, 422–425.

Schall, B. (1988). Olfaction in infants and children: Developmental and functional perspectives. *Chemical Senses, 13*, 145–190.

Schmidt, A., Hammann, F., Wölnerhanssen, B., Meyer-Gerspach, A.C., Drewe, J.,

Beglinger, C., Borgwardt, S. (2014). Green tea extract enhances parieto-frontal connectivity during working memory processing. *Psychopharmacology (Berlin)*, 231(19):3879–88. doi: 10.1007/s00213-014-3526-1. Epub 2014 Mar 19.

Seyle, H. (1973). The evolution of the stress concept: The originator of the concept traces its development from the discovery in 1936 of the alarm reaction to modern therapeutic applications of syntoxic and catatoxic hormones. *American Scientist, 61*, 692–699.

Shinichi K., Atsushi H., Kaori O., Taichi S., Toshifumi M., Satoru E., Shuichi A., Ryoichi N., Hiroyuki A., and Ichiro T. (2006). Green tea consumption and cognitive function: A cross-sectional study from the Tsurugaya Project. *American Journal of Clinical Nutrition*, vol. 83 no. 2, p.355-361.

Shreeve, J. (2015). Beyond the brain [online]. *National Geographic*. Retrieved from http://science.nationalgeographic.com/science/health-and-human-body/human-body/mind-brain/#page=1

Siegel, J. M. (2005). Clues to the functions of mammalian sleep. *Nature, 437,* 1264–1271.

Siegel, J. M. (2009). Sleep viewed as a state of adaptive inactivity. *Nature Reviews Neuroscience, 10,* 747–753.

Silberstein, S. D., Lipton, R. B., & Goadsby, P. J. (2002). *Headache in clinical practice* (2nd ed.). London: Martin Dirnitz.

Silverman, M. J. (2003). Music therapy and clients who are chemically dependent: A review of literature and pilot study. *Arts in Psychotherapy, 30,* 273–281.

Sisk, C. L., & Zehr, J. L. (2005). Pubertal hormones organize the adolescent brain and behavior. *Frontiers in Neuroendocrinology, 26,* 163–174.

Song, H. J., Seo, H.-J., Lee, H., Son, H., Choi, S. M., & Lee, S. (2015). Effect of self-acupressure for symptom management: A systematic review. *Complementary Therapies in Medicine, 23,* 68–78.

Spence, D.W., Kayumov, M. A. L., Chen, A., Lowe, A., Jain, U., Katzman, M. A., Shen, J., Perelman, B., Shapiro, C. M. (2004). Acupuncture increases nocturnal melatonin secretion and reduces insomnia and anxiety: a preliminary report. *The Journal of Neuropsychiatry & Clinical Neurosciences.* 16(1), 19–28.

Spink, S. (2002, January). Adolescent brains are works in progress. Inside the Teenage Brain, *Frontline*. Retrieved from http://www.pbs.org/wgbh/pages/frontline/shows/teenbrain/work/adolescent.html

Steptoe, A., Gibson, E. L., Vuononvirta, R., Williams, E. D., Hamer, M., Rycroft, J. A., Erusalimsky, J. D., & Wardle, J. (2007). The effects of tea on psychophysiological stress responsivity and post-stress recovery: A randomised double-blind trial. *Psychopharmacology* (Berlin), *190*(1), 81–89.

Stores, G. (2009). Aspects of sleep disorders in children and adolescents. *Dialogues in Clinical Neuroscience, 11,* 81–90.

Striege, L., Kang, B., Pilkenton, S. J., Rychlik, M., & Apostolidis, M. (2015, February 12). Effect of black tea and black tea pomace polyphenols on α-glucosidase and α-amylase inhibition, relevant to type 2 diabetes prevention. *Frontiers in Nutrition.*

Strous, R. D., & Shoenfeld, Y. (2006). To smell the immune system: Olfaction, autoimmunity and brain involvement. *Autoimmunity Reviews, 6,* 54–60.

Stux, G., Berman, B., & Pomeranz, B. (2000). *Basics of acupuncture* (5th rev. ed.). Heidelberg: Springer.

Susan G. Komen. (2015). Acupressure: What is it? Retrieved from http://ww5.komen.org/BreastCancer/Acupressure.html

Sussman, S., Skara, S., & Ames, S. L. (2008). Substance abuse among adolescents. *Substance Use and Misuse, 43*, 1802–1828.

Swanson, J. M., Kinsbourne, M., Nigg, J., Lanphear, B., Stefanatos, G. A., Volkow, N., et al. (2007). Etiologic subtypes of attention-deficit/hyperactivity disorder: Brain imaging, molecular genetic and environmental factors and the dopamine hypothesis. *Neuropsychology Review, 17*, 39–59.

Takahashi, M., Li, W., Koike, K., et al. (2010). Clinical effectiveness of KSS formula, a traditional folk remedy for alcohol hangover symptoms. *Journal of Natural Medicines*, 64:487–91.

Tartakovsky, M. (2008). Depression and anxiety. Psych Central. Retrieved from http://psychcentral.com/lib/depression-and-anxiety-among-college-students/

ter Wolbeek, M., van Doornen, L. J. P., Kavelaars, A., & Heijnen, C. J. (2006). Severe fatigue in adolescents: A common phenomenon? *Pediatrics, 117*, e1078–e1086.

Thapar, A., Collishaw, S., Potter, R., & Thapar, A. K. (2010). Managing and preventing depression in adolescents. *British Medical Journal, 340*, 254–258.

Thapar, et al. (2012). Depression in adolescence. *Lancet*, 379, 1056–1067.

Thompson, J. J., & Nichter, M. (2011). Complementary and alternative medicine in the US health insurance reform debate: An anthropological assessment is warranted. Society for Medical Anthropology. Retrieved from http://www.medanthro.net/research/cagh/insurancestatements/Thompson&Nichter(CAM).pdf

Ulett, G. A., Han, J., & Han, S. (1998). Traditional and evidence-based acupuncture: History, mechanisms, and present status. *Southern Medical Journal, 91*, 1115–1120.

Ulrich, L. T. (1990). *A midwife's tale: The life of Martha Ballard, based on her diary, 1785–1812.* New York: Knopf.

University of Texas at Austin. (2011, May 19). Mammals first evolved big brains for better sense of smell. *UT News*. Retrieved from http://www.utexas.edu/news/2011/05/19/geosciences_rowe_smell/

U.S. Department of Agriculture and U.S. Department of Health and Human Services. (2010). *Dietary guidelines for Americans* (7th ed.). Washington, DC: U.S. Government Printing Office.

Valnet, J. (1982). *A practice of aromatherapy: A classic compendium of plant medicines and their healing properties.* Rochester, VT: Healing Arts Press.

Varney, E., & Buckle, J. (2013) Effect of inhaled essential oils on mental exhaustion and moderate burnout: a small pilot study. *Journal of Alternative and Complementary Medicine*, 19(1):69–71.

Vinson, J. A., Teufel, K., & Wu, N. (2004). Green and black teas inhibit atherosclerosis by lipid, antioxidant, and fibrinolytic mechanisms. *Journal of Agricultural and Food Chemistry, 52*(11), 3661–3665.

Walls, D. (2009). Herbs and natural therapies for pregnancy, birth and breast-feeding. *International Journal of Childbirth Education, 24*, 29–37.

Wang, S., Fuh, J. L., Lu, S. R., & Juang, K. D. (2006). Chronic daily headache in adolescents. *Neurology, 66*, 193–197.

WebMD. (2014). What are REM and non-REM sleep? Retrieved from http://www.webmd.com/sleep-disorders/guide/sleep-101

WebMD. (2015). Relaxation techniques for migraines and headaches. Retrieved from http://www.webmd.com/migraines-headaches/guide/relaxation-techniques

Weimer, K., Schulte, J., Maichle, A., et al. (2012). Effects of ginger and expectations on symptoms of nausea in a balanced placebo design. *Public Library of Science*, 7(11):e49031.

Welsh, C. (1997). Touch with oils: A pertinent part of holistic hospice care. *American Journal of Hospice and Palliative Care, 14*(January/February), 42–44.

Williams, C., & Garland, A. (2002). Identifying and challenging unhelpful thinking. *Advances in Psychiatric Treatment, 8*, 377–386.

Witkiewitz, K., & Marlatt, G. A. (2005). Mindfulness-based relapse prevention for alcohol and substance use disorders. *Journal of Cognitive Psychotherapy: An International Quarterly, 19*, 211–220.

Wu, Y., Zhang, Y., Xie, G., Zhao, A., Pan, X., Chen, T., et al. (2012, September). The metabolic responses to aerial diffusion of essential oils. *PLOS ONE, 7*, 1–11.

Yoga.org.nz. (2015). Definition of yoga. Retrieved from http://yoga.org.nz/what-is-yoga/yoga_definition.htm

Zeidan, F., Lobanov, O., Hadsel, M., Martucci, K., Quevedo, A., Starr, C., et al. (2014). Brain structure shows who is most sensitive to pain. Wake Forest Baptist Medical Center. Retrieved from http://www.wakehealth.edu/News-Releases/2014/Brain_Structure_Shows_Who_is_Most_Sensitive_to_Pain.htm

Index

//////////////

Note: Italicized page locators refer to illustrations.